ANATOMY
COLORING BOOK
1ST EDITION

"THE MOST BEAUTIFUL EXPERIENCE WE CAN HAVE IS THE
MYSTERIOUS. IT IS THE FUNDAMENTAL EMOTION THAT STANDS AT
THE CRADLE OF TRUE ART AND TRUE SCIENCE."
ALBERT EINSTEIN, THE WORLD AS I SEE IT

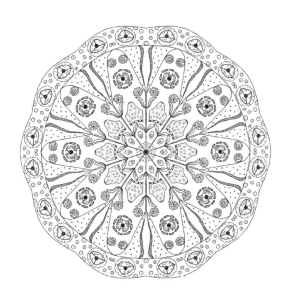

GARY HEMMINGS, BA(HONS), MA, PGCE.

ABOUT THE AUTHOR

Gary Hemmings is a teacher, writer and designer with degrees in the Arts and Humanities. He is currently studying for a science degree with the Open University, and somehow finds the time to do so whilst teaching, caring for his teenage twins and immersing himself in the world of print-on-demand publishing. His loves are his family, the mountains and learning.

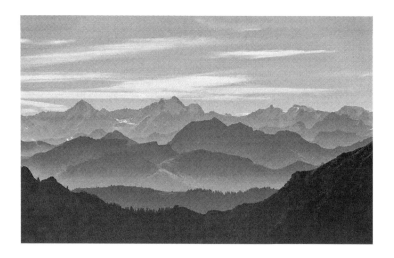

TABLE OF CONTENTS

CELLS
EUKARYOTIC CELLS, NUCLEUS, CHROMOSOMES, MITOCHONDRIA, RIBOSOMES, ROUGH AND SMOOTH ENDOPLASMIC RETICULUM, LYSOSOMES, GOLGI APPARATUS, TYPES OF CELL, MITOSIS.

TISSUE
EPITHELIAL, MUSCLE, CONNECTIVE, NERVE

SKELETAL SYSTEM
THORAX, LONG BONE, CARTILAGE, PELVIC GIRDLE, UPPER LIMBS, TARSALS,CARPALS, SKULL

ORGANS
HEART, LUNGS, RESPIRATORY SYSTEM, ABDOMINAL ORGANS, LARGE INTESTINE, SMALL INTESTINE, LIVER, PANCREAS, KIDNEY

THE BRAIN
NEURONS, BRAIN, CRANIAL NERVES, SPINAL COLUMN AND CORD, SYNAPSE AND SEROTONIN.

THE SENSES
TOUCH, TASTE, SMELL, HEARING, SIGHT.

The Cell

"What you are - what each of us is - is an assemblage of roughly a trillion cells, of thousands of different sorts. Most of these cells are "daughters" of the egg and sperm cell whose union started you... and not a single one of the cells that compose you knows who you are, or cares."

Daniel C Dennett, We Earth Neurons, 1999.

Though this may be true, it is certainly not the case that people do not care - people care, they care a lot. They care enough to ask questions; they care enough to seek answers; they care enough to devise and design solutions to all the problems they encounter, large and small. Those assemblages of cells, when taken as a whole, care enough to beautify the world in which they live, to add colour and contour to the shape of the lives they form. It is a strange thing indeed. The cells do not care, and yet, if we cast aside the microscope for a moment, if we imagine Robert Hooke had not, in 1665, revealed the infinitesimal realm of ourselves to us, then we cease to be assemblages and return to being entire, caring, compassionate, conscious souls. Hooke showed us the truth, yet somehow our cells still carry a mystery within themselves - the mystery of our better nature.

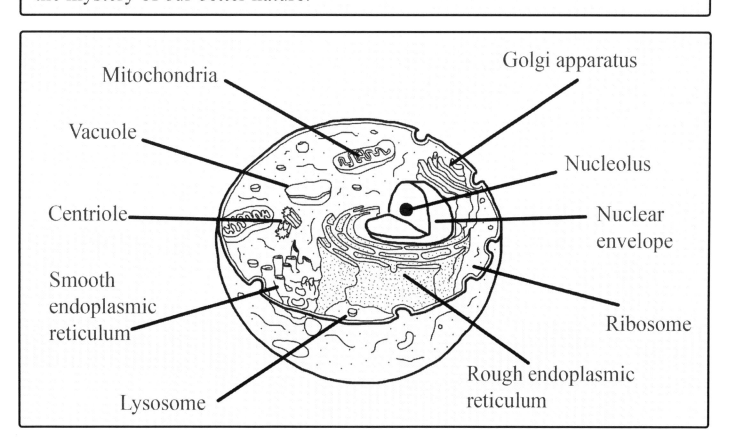

<u>Notes</u>

_____
_____
_____
_____
_____
_____
_____
_____
_____
_____
_____
_____
_____
_____
_____
_____
_____
_____
_____
_____

Color Key:

NUCLEUS, NUCLEOLUS, ENDOPLASMIC RETICULUM, GOLGI APPARATUS, MITOCHONDRIA, RIBOSOME, CYTOPLASM, MICROTUBULES

(Due to size, some cell components are missing from the diagram)

Eukaryotic Cell

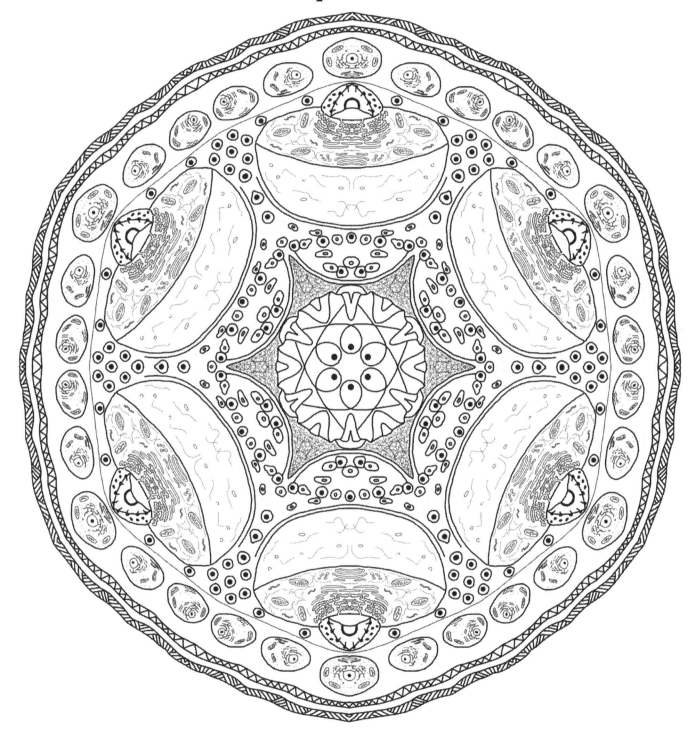

The Nucleus

"In our every cell, furled at the nucleus, there is a ribbon two yards long and just ten atoms wide. Over a hundred million miles of DNA in every human individual, enough to wrap five million times around our world and make the Midgard serpent blush for shame, make even the ourobouros worm swallow hard in disbelief."

Alan Moore, Snakes and Ladders, 2001

The nucleus of the cell is a membrane bound organelle formed from an impermeable nuclear envelope and an inner matrix, which provides the nucleus with a definite shape. It contains almost the entire genome of the organism packaged up as chromosomes; chromosomes are made from the double helix spiral of the DNA molecules mentioned above and they provide the blueprint for all the proteins that give shape and form to life. The cell nucleus, therefore, is of vital importance to the existence of life on Earth. It is both Fort Knox and the Great Library of Alexandria, and deep within its centre can be found the nucleolus, a membraneless structure made from rDNA, the DNA that codes for ribosomal rRNA.

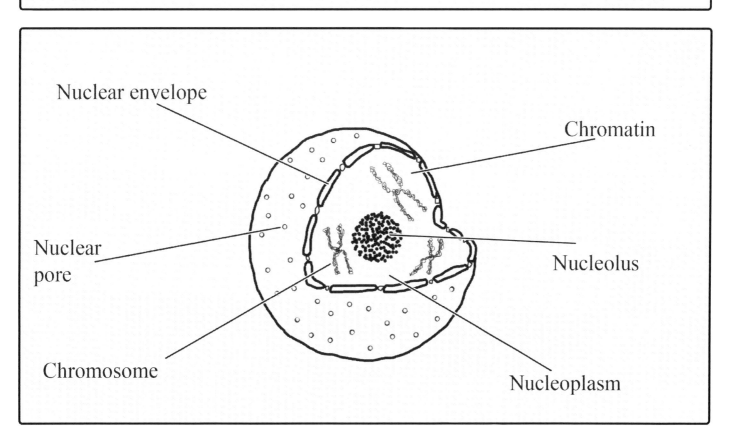

Notes

_____

_____

_____

_____

_____

_____

_____

_____

_____

_____

_____

_____

_____

_____

_____

_____

_____

_____

_____

_____

_____

_____

Color Key:

NUCLEUR MEMBRANE
NUCLEUR PORES
DNA
NUCLEOLUS

Nucleus

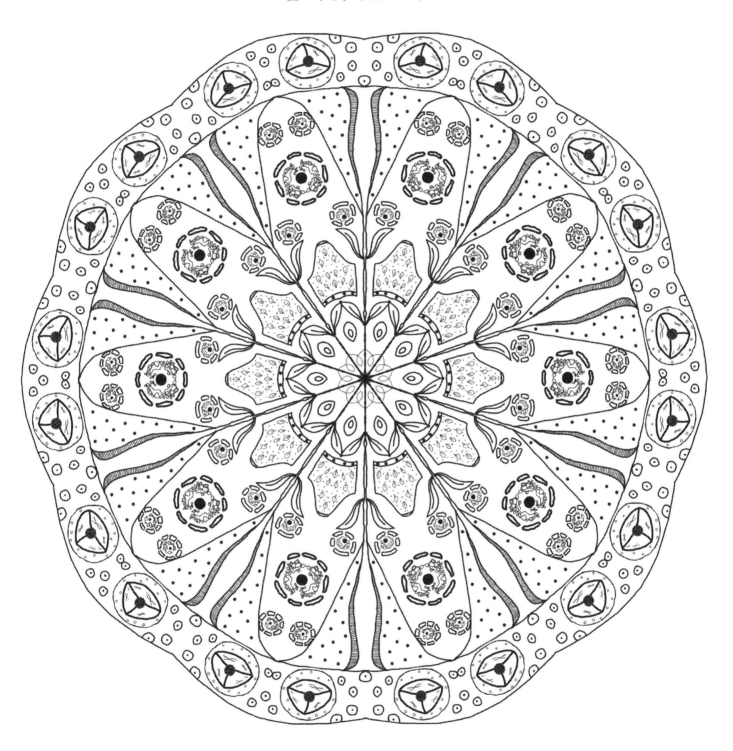

Chromosomes

"[After science lost] its mystical inspiration... man's destiny was no longer determined from "above" by a super-human wisdom and will, but from "below" by the sub-human agencies of glands, genes, atoms, or waves of probability... A puppet of the Gods is a tragic figure, a puppet suspended on his chromosomes is merely grotesque."

Arthur Koestler, The Sleepwalkers, 1959

Although the cells within different species can be almost indistinguishable, assuming them to be of the same type - human, mouse and pig heart cells, for instance - the chromosomes contained within the nucleus of the cells will be vastly different. Different in number and different in the arrangement, or pattern, of their nucleotides. The chromosomes generally appear in pairs and carry the genetic recipe particular to the organism, furled and folded into its distinct lobes. Such is the miracle of this compaction that human chromosome 1, the longest chromosome in humans, is 125 million nucleotide rungs in length and spans 8.5cm. That's 8.5 cm crammed into a single chromosome; across all 46 chromosomes in humans you have over 2 metres of DNA in total in every single cell. Now, that's a lot of silly string on which to hang a puppet.

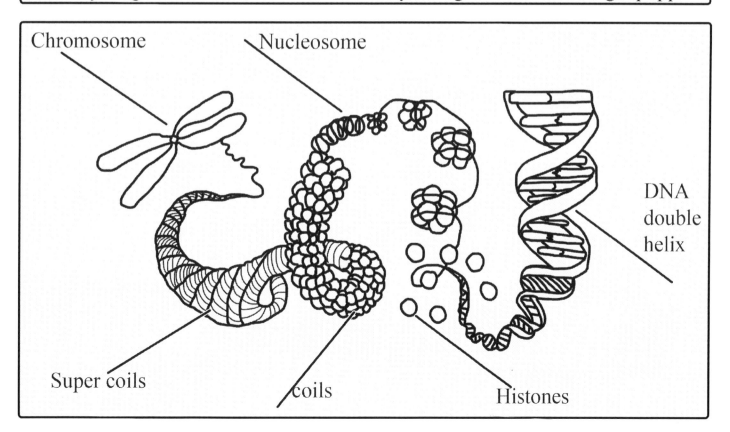

<u>Notes</u>

Color Key:

CHROMOSOME, CHROMATIN LOOP, NUCELOSOMES, DNA DOUBLE HELIX.

NUCLEOBASES: GUANINE, CYTOSINE, ADENINE, THYMINE

Chromosomes

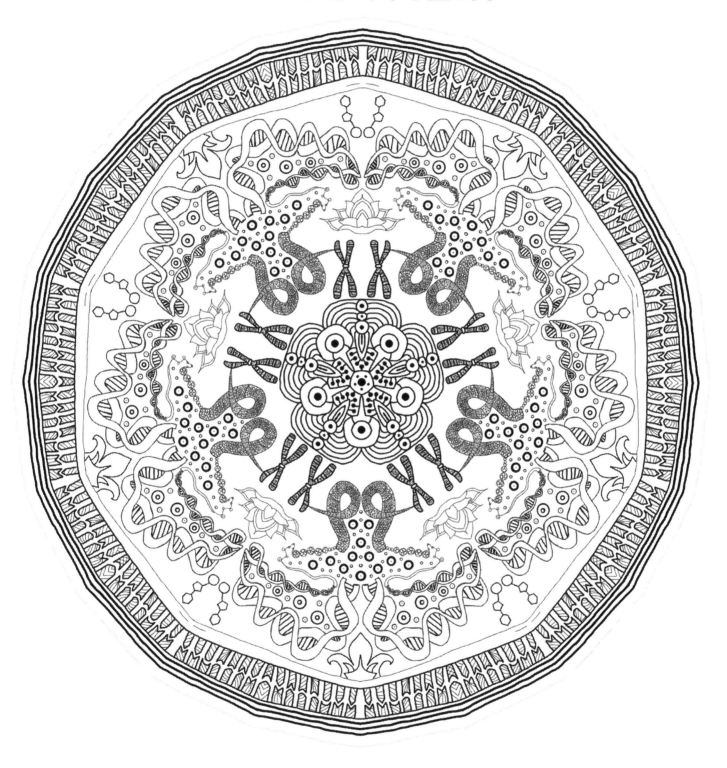

Mitochondria

"My mitochondria comprise a very large proportion of me. I cannot do the calculation, but I suppose there is as much of them in sheer dry bulk as there is the rest of me. Looked at in this way, I could be taken for a very large, motile colony of respiring bacteria, operating a complex system of nuclei, microtubules and neurons for the pleasure and sustenance of their family, and running, at the moment, a typewriter."

Lewis Thomas, A Long Line of Cells: Collected essay,s, 1990

Mitochondria are the powerhouse of the cell, supplying and regulating the delivery of energy through the repeated hydrolysis of the chemical adenosine triphosphate (ATP). They are also carriers of their own chromosomes, passed down the maternal line of inheritance - the term mitochondrial Eve is often used to suggest the most recent common ancestor of all humans - the mother of the human race. Most unusual of all, however, is the fact that mitochondria are thought to be the result of an anciet eukaryotic cell engulfing a prokaryote. The successful symbiotic relationship that developed means that you carry within every one of your cells a descendent of an alien bacteria.

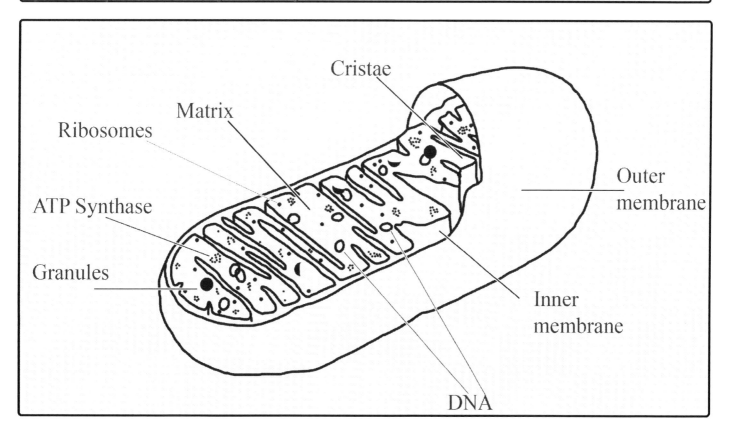

Notes

_____
_____
_____
_____
_____
_____
_____
_____
_____
_____
_____
_____
_____
_____
_____
_____
_____
_____
_____
_____
_____
_____
_____

Color Key:

OUTER MEMBRANE

INNER MEMBRANE

MATRIX

(Smaller components may be difficult to colour but include: granules, mitochondrial DNA and ATP synthase particles)

Mitochondria

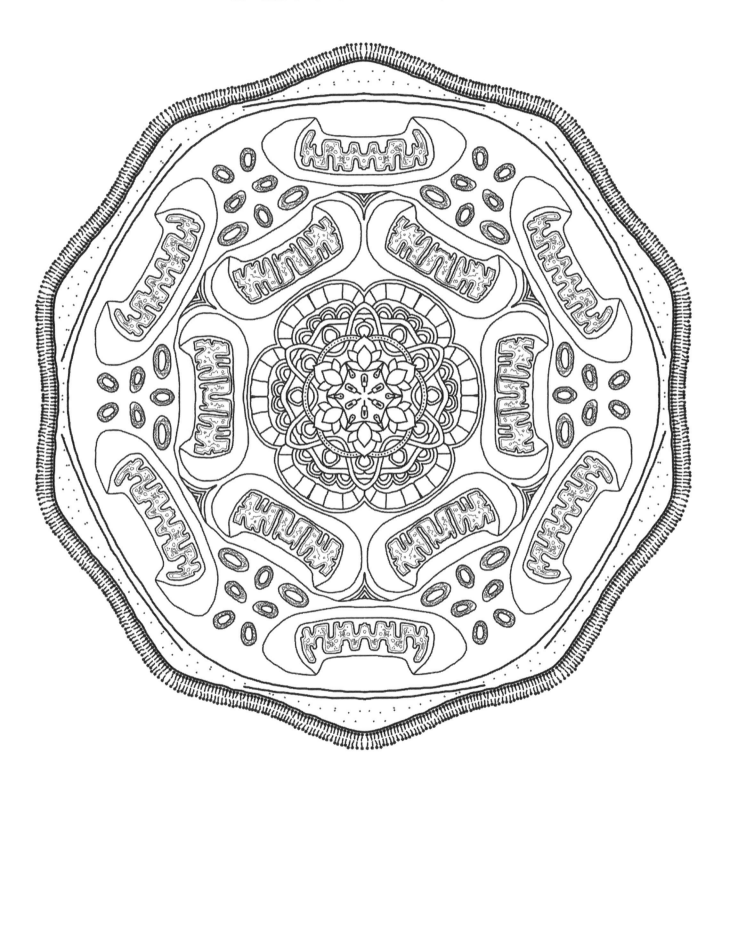

Ribosomes

"Ricin is classed as a ribosone inhibiting protein, which is abbreviated to RIP"
Kathryn Harkup, A is for Arsenic: The
Poisons of Agatha Christie, 2015.

Ribosomes are protein making machines. In a single mammalian cell there may be an astonishing 10 million ribosomes, floating free in the cytoplasm or integrated into the rough endoplasmic reticulum. They are formed from two subunits and are ephemeral in nature; once they have completed the task of assembling a polypeptide chain they break apart and are either recycled or dissolved. By translating the codons of a mRNA chain, ribosomes can select amino acids and join them together at a rate of 200 per minute. The larger sub-unit plays a catalytic role in this process, whereas the small sub-unit takes the role of translator.

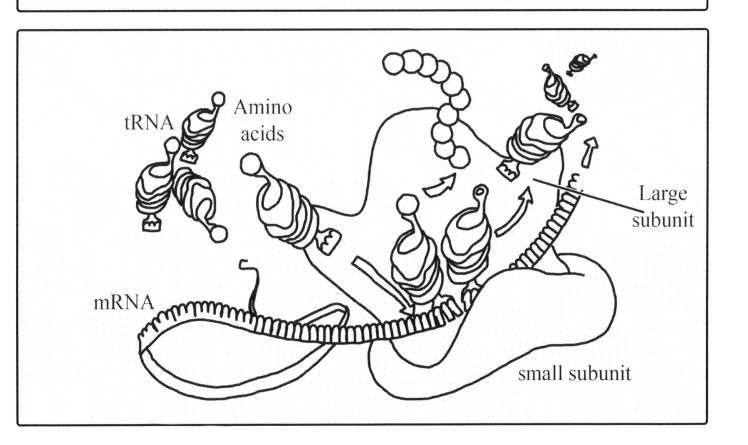

<u>Notes</u>

Color Key:

Ribosomes

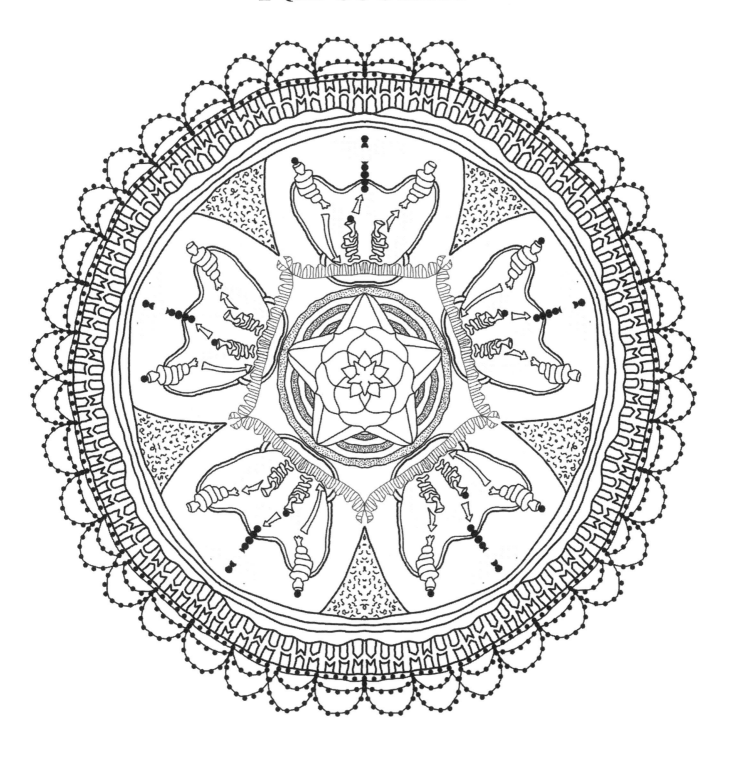

Rough and Smooth Endoplasmic Reticulum

"Is it not love that knows how to make smooth things rough and rough things smooth?"

Vikram Seth, An Equal Music, 1999

Endoplasmic reticulum is a network of membranes that occupy approximately 10% of the total cell volume. The two types differ in appearance and function: rough endoplasmic reticulum (RER) is formed from folds of cytosol and is studded with countless ribosomes, which attach to the sides and produce proteins whilst the RER acts like a quality control unit; smooth endoplasmic reticulum (SER) is abundant in liver cells, is more tubular, like a hydrothermal vent, and is integral to the production of lipids, phospholipids and steroids, whilst also being involved in the metabolism of carbohydrates. One of the tasks of the SER in the liver is the detoxification of alcohol and barbituates, and it is in the course of this task that it can double its surface area to better absorb the chemicals.

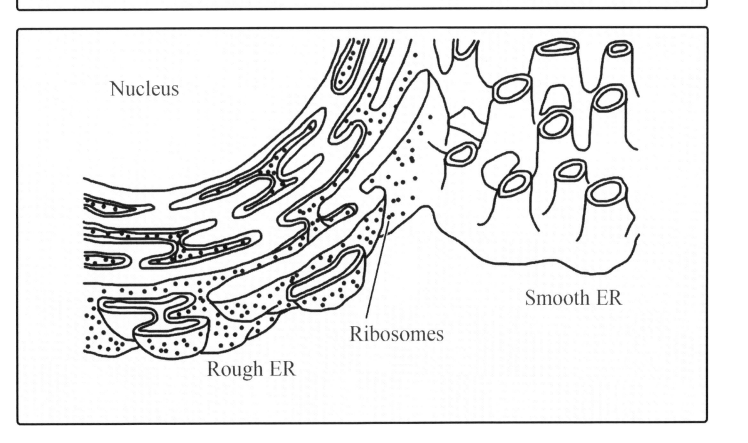

Nucleus

Smooth ER

Ribosomes

Rough ER

Notes

_____

_____

_____

_____

_____

_____

_____

_____

_____

_____

_____

_____

_____

_____

_____

_____

_____

_____

_____

_____

Color Key:

ROUGH ENDOPLASMIC RETICULUM
RIBOSOMES (DOTS)
CISTERNAE AND CISTERNAL SPACE

SMOOTH ENDOPLSMIC RETICULUM

Rough & Smooth
Endoplasmic Reticulum

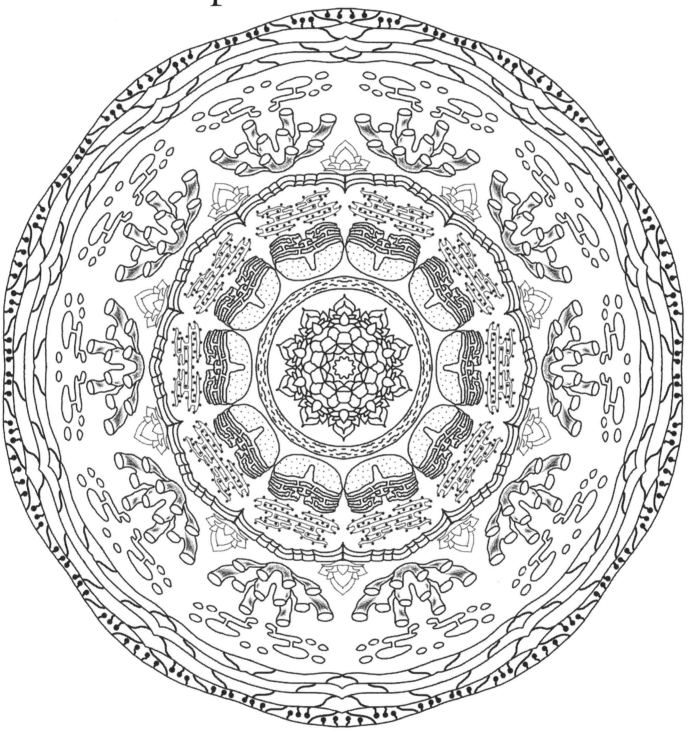

Lysosomes

"The possibility that lysosomes might accidentally become ruptured under certain conditions, and kill or injure their host-cells as a result, was considered right after we got our first clues to the existence of these particles."

Christian de Duve, Nobel Lecture, 1974

This image of the lysosome as a sac of apocalyptic potential gives a clue to just exactly what Duve discovered hidden inside cells. However, what was once thought of as the trash can of the cell, a waste disposal unit brimming with destructive enzymes and acids whose sole purpose is to digest and recycle proteins and cellular components in a process termed autophagy, is now thought of a decision-making centre that controls the rate of growth. Lysosomes are more akin to a control switch that can determine whether the resources are available for growth, or whether an excess of something needs breaking down. They play an important role in regulating the life of an organism and have been shown to prolong cell life rather than curtail it.

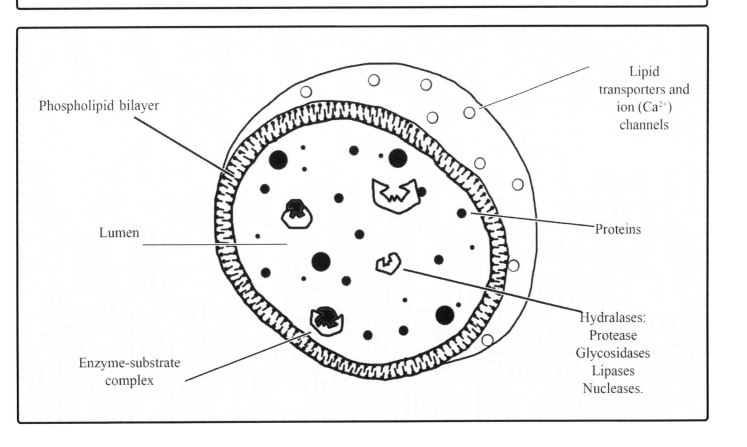

<u>Notes</u>

_____
_____
_____
_____
_____
_____
_____
_____
_____
_____
_____
_____
_____
_____
_____
_____
_____
_____
_____
_____
_____
_____
_____

Color Key:

MEMBRANE

GLYCOSYLATED MEMBRANE TRANSPORT PROTEINS

LIPID LAYER

HYDROLYTIC ENZYME MIXTURE

Lysosome

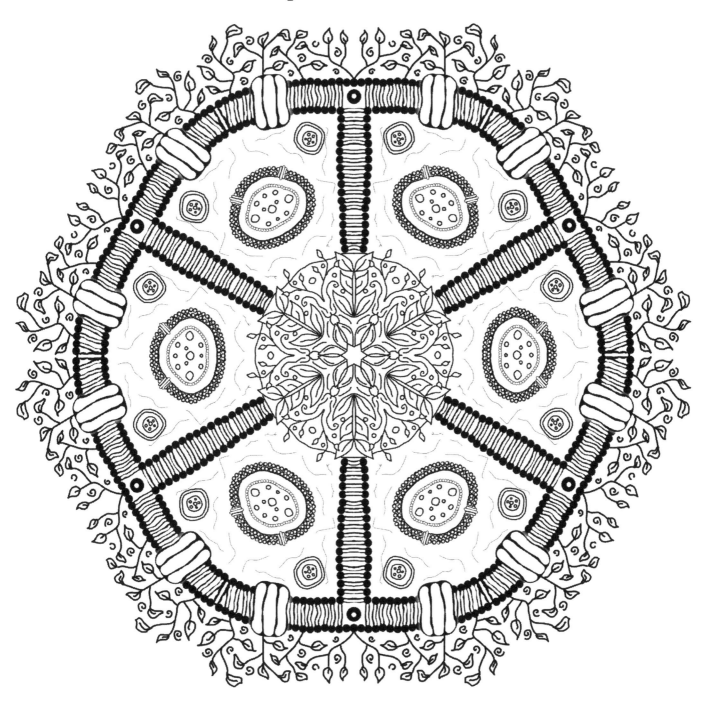

The Golgi Apparatus

"Owl," said Rabbit shortly, "you and I have brains. The others have fluff. If there is any thinking to be done in this forest - and when I say thinking I mean thinking - you and I must do it."

A. A. Milne, The House at Pooh Corner.

The Golgi apparatus was discovered by Camillo Golgi in 1898, after staining the cerebellum of an owl with osmium dichromate. It has come to be recognised as a sorting and transport centre for proteins, delivering them in packages to the plasma membrane and other destinations in the cell. Proteins arrive in vesicles, are processed in the cisternae of the golgi and sorted into golgi vesicles for secretion or storage. As the process ensues, each cisterna progresses through the stack, much like a dimishing heap of maple syrup coated pancakes. Cells that produce secretions, such as enzyme producing pancreatic cells, have particularly well-developed golgi apparatus.

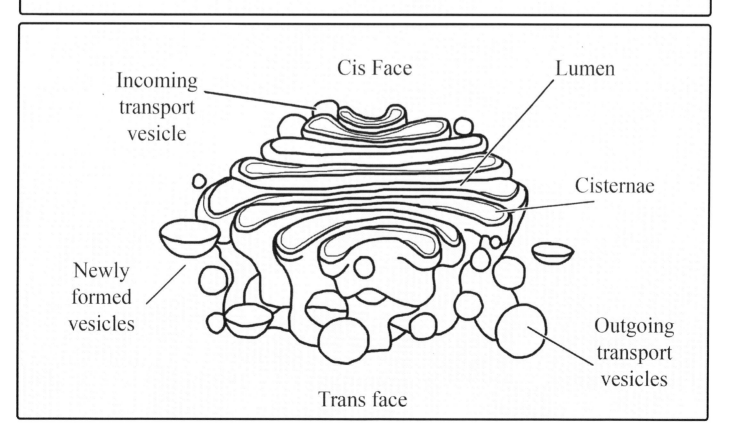

<u>Notes</u>

Color Key:

CISTERNAE
LUMEN
INCOMING TRANSPORT VESICLE
NEWLY FORMING VESICLE

Golgi Apparatus

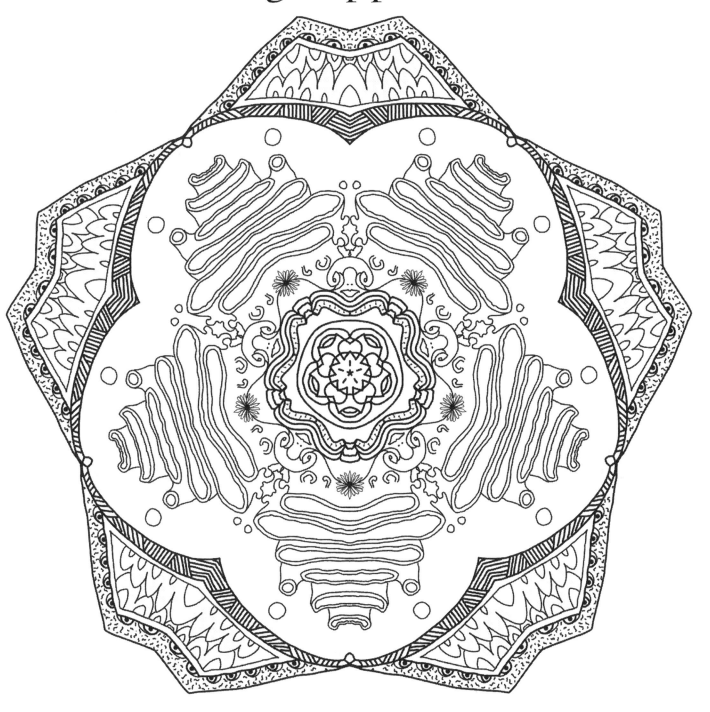

Cell Types

"It is incredible to think that mammalian cells carry about 20,000 genes, and yet it only takes four to turn a fully differentiated cell into something that is pluripotent"

Nessa Carey, The Epigentics Revolution, 2011

Although the cells of the body all contain the entire genome locked inside their nucleus, the cells of a complex organism are differentiated for their function. A heart cell is different in shape and nature to a kidney cell or a skin cell, and so on. So, we have the same blueprint as determined by the DNA but a different form emergent as a result of gene expression. The model of the cell shown earlier in the book is an ideal model, conceived to convey the various organelles found enclosed within the membrane; it is a version of the truth, but not the entire truth. For example, within the brain only a fraction of the cells take the form and function of neurons, the remainder of the brain is an assortment of glia, blood and endothelial cells. All cells differentiate at the stage of foetal development from embryonic stem cells. These are described as pluripotent as they have the ability to become any cell type.

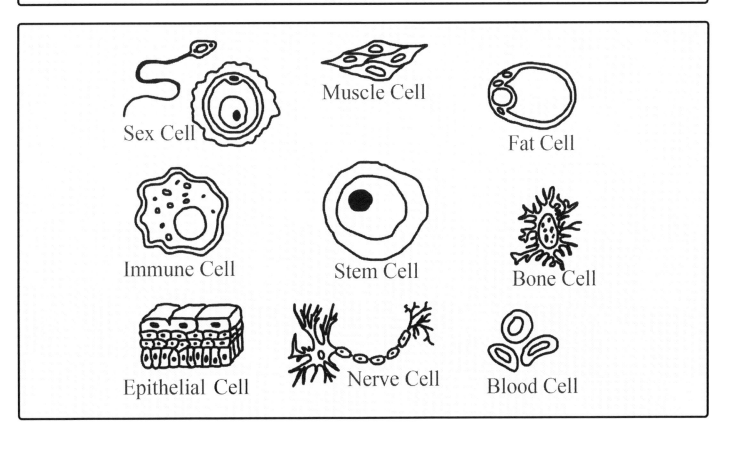

Notes

Cell Types

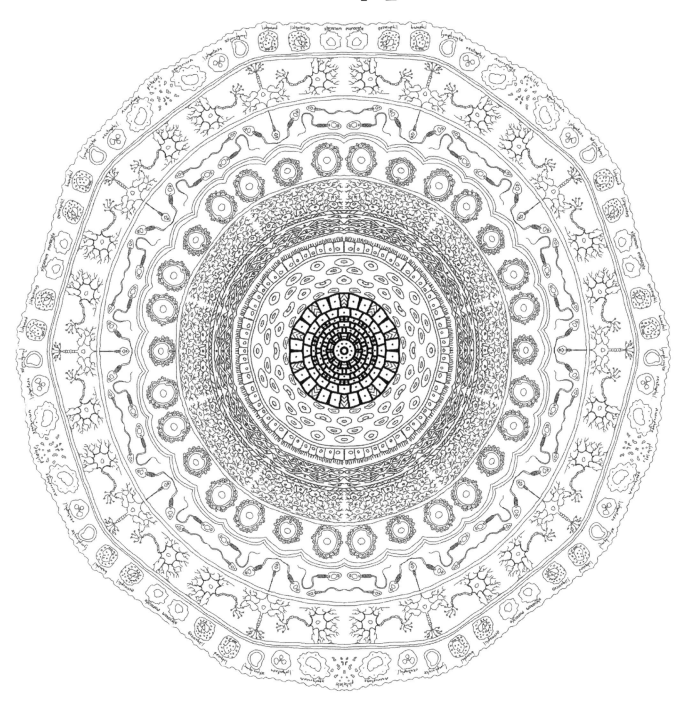

Epithelial Tissue

"Eighty percent of cancers, known as carcinomas, arise in epithelial cells - that is the cells that make up the skin and linings of organs. Breast cancers, for instance, don't just grow randomly within the breast, but normally begin in the milk ducts."

Bill Bryson, The Body: A Guide for Occupants, 2019

Epithelial tissue has no blood supply but recieves its oxygen through the basal layer. The cells are tightly packed together and serve to protect the body by creating a barrier, as well as being involved in secretion and absorption. The shape of epithelial cells vary and are denoted as squamous, cuboidal, columnar and transitional. Where the cells are stratified across a number of layers the uppermost layer is used to define the tissue. The diferent types of epithelial tissue are adapted for different functions and can be found in different organ systems. For example, simple squamous tissue allows diffusion and is therefore found in the lungs; simple cuboidal and columnar enable absorption and secretion and are found in the GI tract.

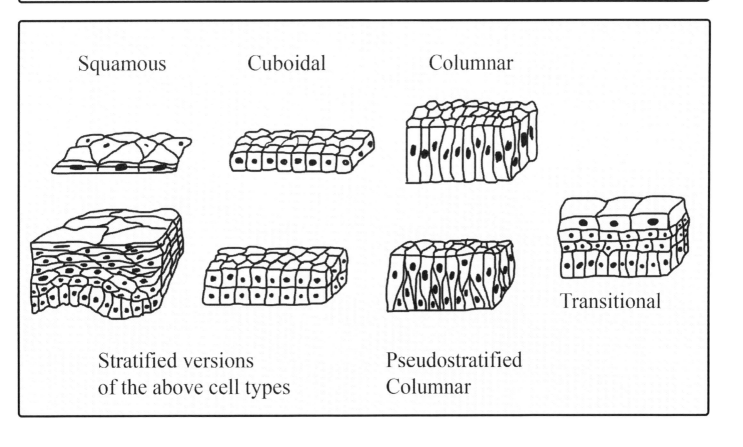

Squamous   Cuboidal   Columnar

Transitional

Stratified versions
of the above cell types

Pseudostratified
Columnar

Notes

_____
_____
_____
_____
_____
_____
_____
_____
_____
_____
_____
_____
_____
_____
_____
_____
_____
_____
_____
_____

Color Key:

SQUAMOUS
CUBOIDAL
COLUMNAR
PSEUDOSTRATIFIED
STRATIFIED SQUAMOUS
GLANDULAR EPITHELIUM:
EXOCRINE, ENDOCRINE.

EPITHELIUM TISSUE

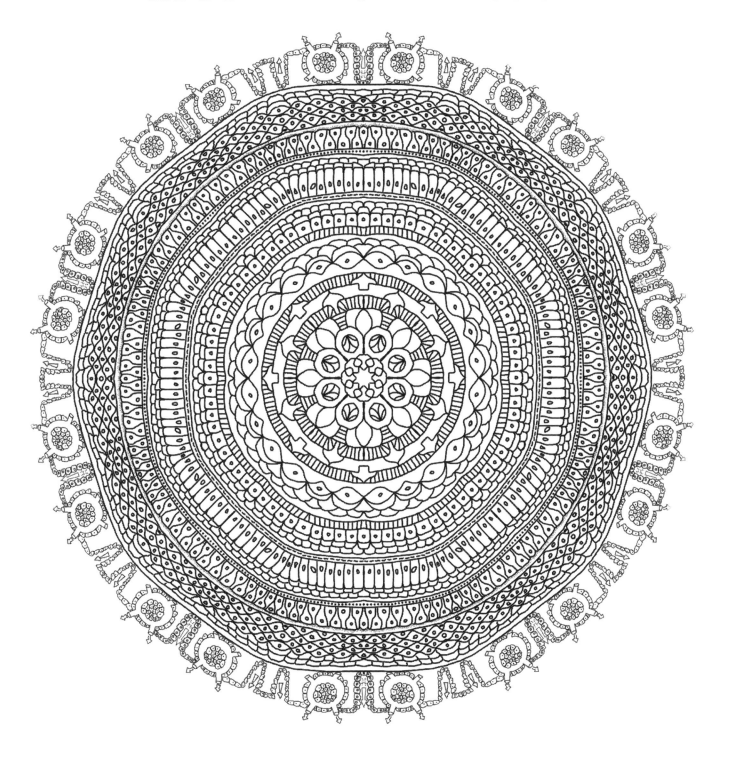

Muscle Tissue

"He was mastered by the sheer surging of life, the tidal wave of being, the perfect joy of each separate muscle, joint and sinew in that it was everything that was not death, that it was aglow and rampant, expressing itself in movement, flying exultantly under the stars."

Jack London, The Call of the Wild, 1903

Muscle is all about contraction and relies on the ability of cells to shorten and thereby enable movement. Muscle tissue is well supplied with oxygen through a network of blood vesels, and this oxygen, along with glucose similarly supplied, enables aerobic respiration to occur. The product of this reaction, ATP, is fundamental to the contraction of muscle fibres, as it passes through a series of chemical changes that alter the shape of the molecule. These changes in shape provide the motor for the cross-bridge cycle, wherein myosin binds to and releases itself from an actin filament within sarcomere sections of the muscle fibre. The resulting ratcheting of the actin filament is how you are able to turn the page , your head and make every rampant movement your heart desires.

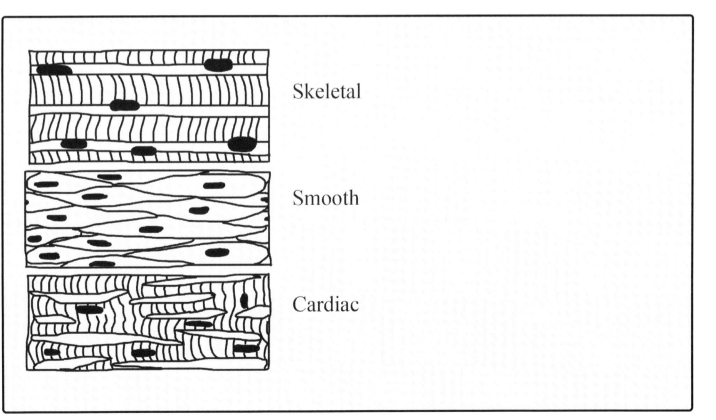

Skeletal

Smooth

Cardiac

Notes

_____

Color Key:

SMOOTH
CARDIAC
SKELETAL

MUSCLE TISSUE

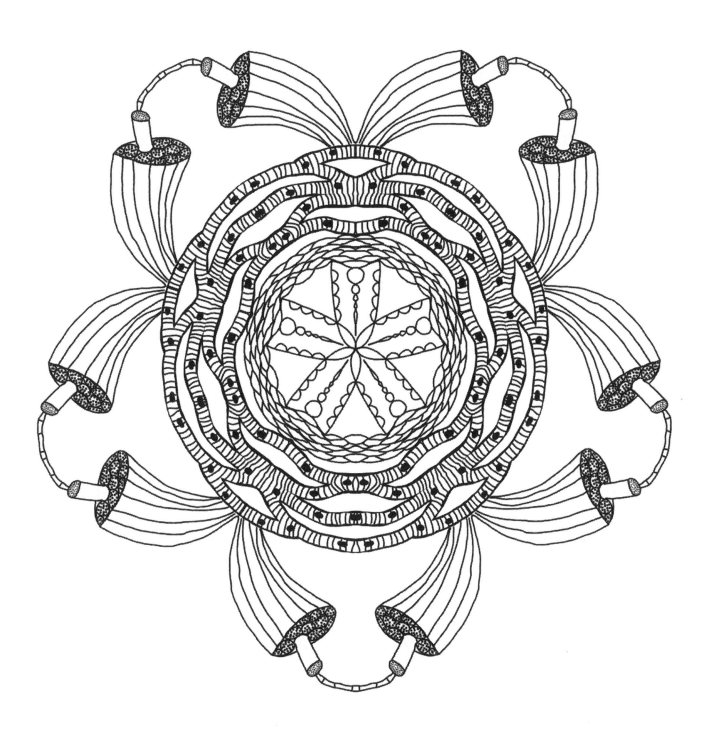

Connective Tissue

"Happiness is not a noun or a verb. It is a conjunction. Connective tissue."
Eric Weiner, The Geography of Bliss, 2008

Connective tissue binds and supports other tissue in the body. The cells within this tissue type are called fibroblasts and these are suspended amongst a fluid matrix which also contain tissue fibres. Loose connective tissue provides support, flexibility and strength to internal organs and blood and lymph vessels and nerves. The dense variety is stronger and thicker as a result of a higher proportion of collagen; it is found predominantly in ligaments and tendons. Adipose tissue stores fat - the less said the better - but has a use in protecting organs and preventing heat loss. Finally, reticular tissue is mesh-like and supports soft organs such as the lymphatic system, the spleen and the liver. It's name comes from the latin for "little net," which, oddly enough, is the root of the name of the gladiator with the trident and fishing net - the retiarius - who, ironically, could gain Caesar's favour by separating the limbs from the body of his opponent.

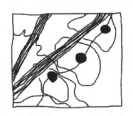

Loose Connective

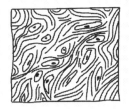

Dense irregular

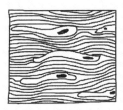

Dense regular

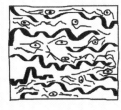

Elastic

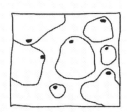

Adipose

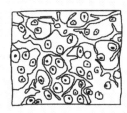

Reticular

Notes

_____
_____
_____
_____
_____
_____
_____
_____
_____
_____
_____
_____
_____
_____
_____
_____
_____
_____
_____
_____
_____

Color Key:

LOOSE CONNECTIVE
RREGULAR CONNECTIVE
DENSE REGULAR CONNECTIVE
ELASTIC CONNECTIVE
ADIPOSE TISSUE
RETICULAR CONNECTIVE

CONNECTIVE TISSUE

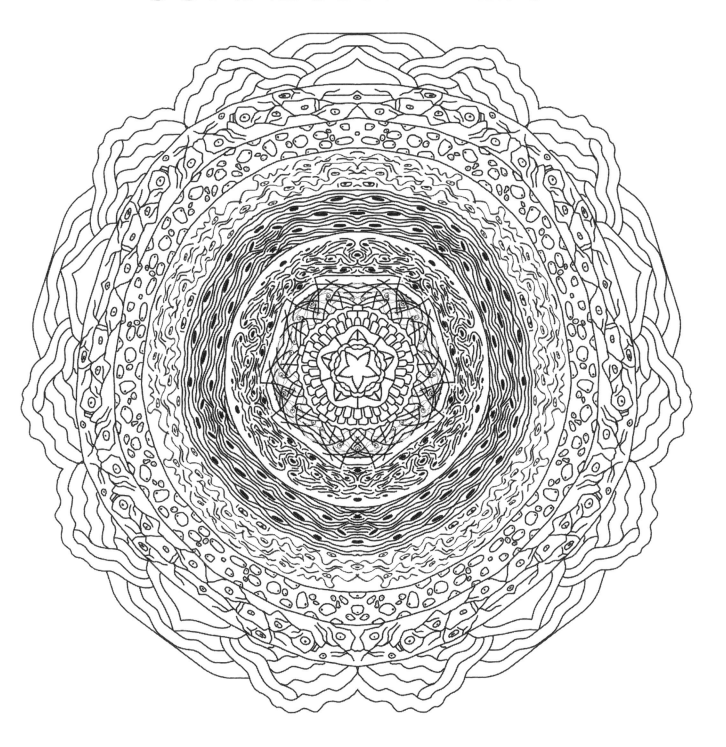

Nervous tissue

"How it is that anything so remarkable as a state of consciousness comes about as a result of irritating nervous tissue, is just as unaccountable as the appearance of the djinn when Aladdin rubbed his lamp in the story."

Thomas Henry Huxley, The Elements of
Physiology and Hygiene, 1868

Nerve tissue is the source of every feeling you have ever experienced. It is the foundation of your senses, the place in which your moral compass sits and the home to all your thoughts and inspirations. It is thanks to Phineas Gage and the awful incident of his being speared through the brain with a tamping rod that we understand the importance of the functioning of nerve tissue to personality. Safe to say, he was never the same again. So, what is nerve tissue? It is formed from impulse carrying nerve cells, which were introduced earlier, and tiny neuroglia, which provide the nerve cells with nutrients. There are three types of neuron, each of which contain axons that send electrochemical signals throughout the Central and peripheral nervous system.

Reflex Arc

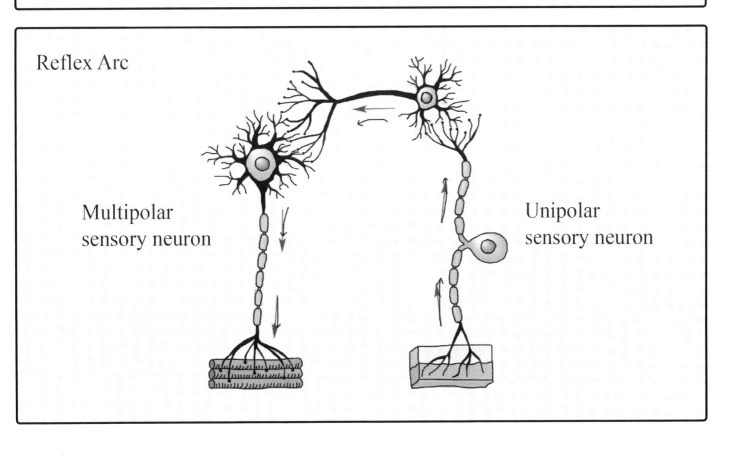

Multipolar
sensory neuron

Unipolar
sensory neuron

Notes

Color Key:

UNIPOLAR NEURON
BIPOLAR NEURON
MULTIPOLAR NEURON
MICROGLIAL CELL

NERVE TISSUE

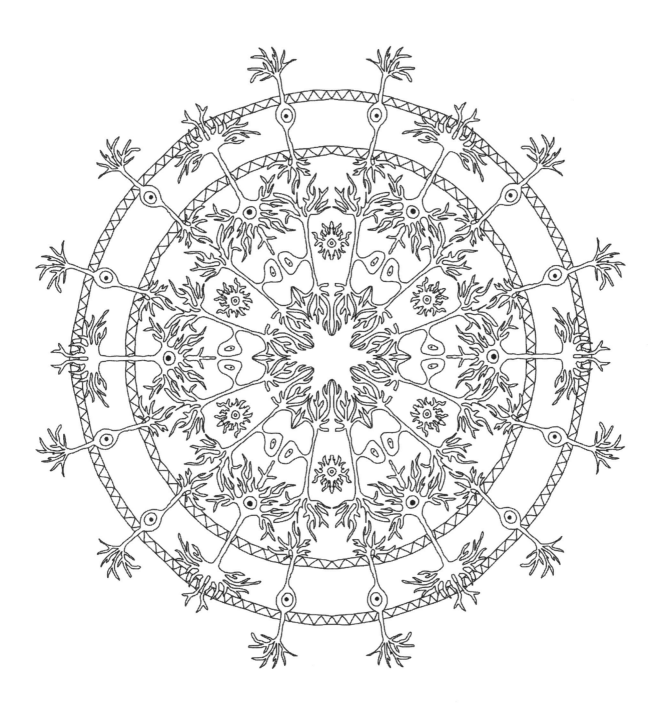

The Bony Thorax

"In 1794, the first clear success in using electricity to restart the heart was recorded by what had become the Royal Humane Society. SophiaGreenhill, a young girl, had fallen from a window in Soho and was pronounced dead by a doctor at Middlesex Hospital. Mr squires, a local member of the society, made it to the girl in around twenty minutes. Using a friction-type electricity machine, he applied shocks to her body. It seemed "in vain", until he began to shock her thorax. Then he felt a pulse, and the child began to breathe again."

Lucy Inglis, Georgian London: Into the Streets, 2012

Much like the thorax of the trilobites of the Cambrian era, the human thorax serves as a protective casing for the vital organs of the body. Housing the heart and lungs, the thorax can be seen as a cage of ribs, numbered 1-12 as they descend from the shoulder: ribs 1-7 are considered "true"; 8-10 "false" - as the costal cartllage joins the rib above; and 11 and 12 "floating" - as they have no anterior attachment point.

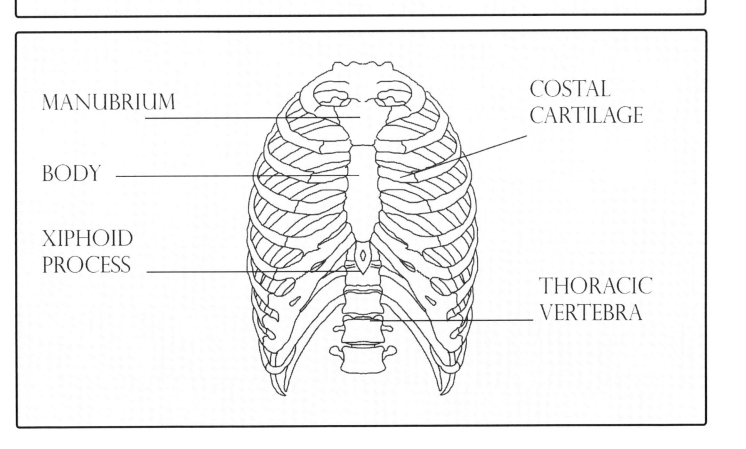

MANUBRIUM

BODY

XIPHOID PROCESS

COSTAL CARTILAGE

THORACIC VERTEBRA

Notes

_____
_____
_____
_____
_____
_____
_____
_____
_____
_____
_____
_____
_____
_____
_____
_____
_____
_____
_____
_____
_____

Color Key:

STERNUM: MANUBRIUM; BODY; XIPHOID PROCESS

RIBS: TRUE; FALSE; FLOATING.

COSTAL CARTLIAGE
THORACIC VERTEBRA

BONY THORAX

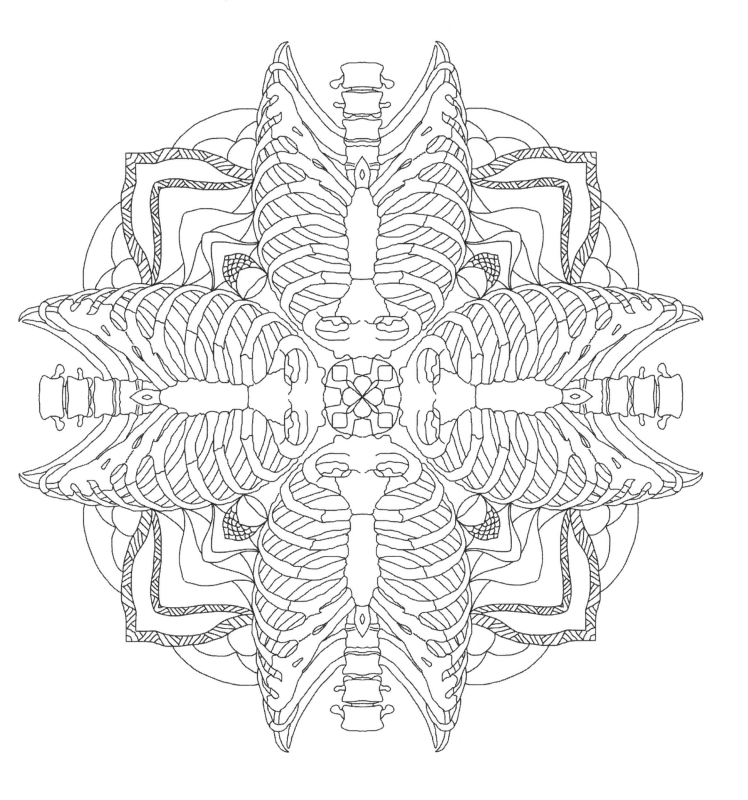

Long Bone

"I will look down and see my murmuring bones and the deep water like wind, like a roof of wind, and after a long time they cannot distinguish even bones upon the lonely and inviolate sand."

William Faulkner, The Sound and the Fury, 1929

The arms and legs of the human body are largely supported by long bones, only the patella and bones of the wrist and ankle are excluded from the catogory. They are longer than they are wide and have two bulbed ends separated by a shaft called the diaphysis. The thick outer layer of compact bone tissue conceals an inner medullary cavity in which bone marrow is found. Bone marrow is identified as being either red or yellow: red marrow contains stem cells capable of becoming red or white blood cells or platelets; yellow bone marrow is largely composed of fat but also contains stem cells that can become cartilage, fat or bone cells. The epiphyseal line within the red bone marrow is a remnant of growth of the bone during childhood.

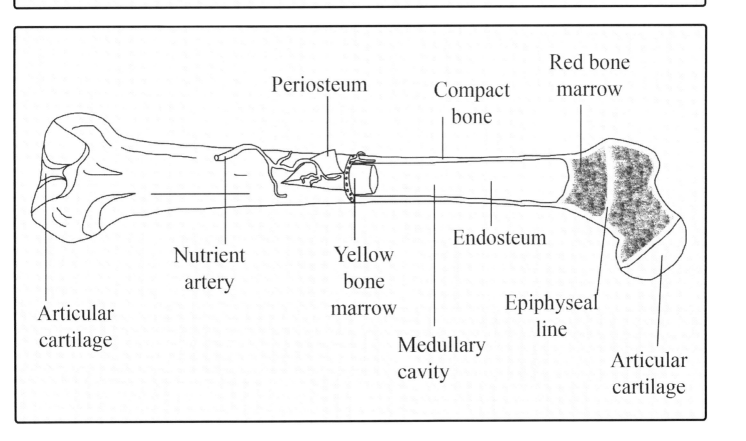

Notes

Color Key:

EPIPHYSIS: ARTICULAR CARTILAGE

DIAPHYSIS: PERIOSTEUM, ENDOSTEUM, MEDULLARY CAVITY

EPIPHYSIS: SPONGY BONE, EPIPHYSEAL LINE, ARTICULAR CARTTILAGE.

Long Bone

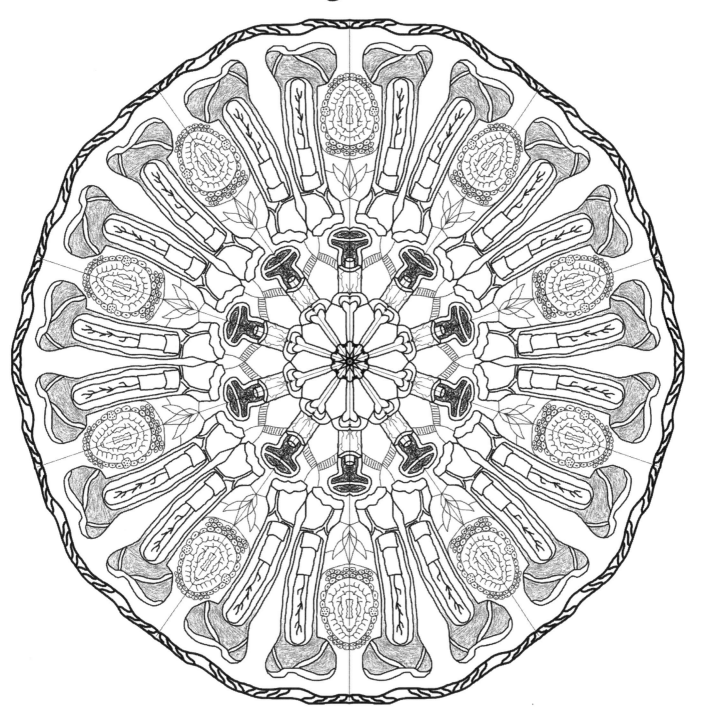

Cartilage

"Use Cod Liver Oil - according to studies, the fatty acids found abundantly in the oil can switch off enzymes that break down cartilage (the smooth protective coating in our bodies)."

C. D. Shelton, Arthritis: Joint Pain, 2014

Cartilage is a form of connective tissue made up of specialist cells called chondrocytes. These cells are highly efficient at producing extracellular matrix composed of collagen, proteoglycan and elastin fibers. As there are no blood vessels in cartilage, nutrients are delivered by diffusion through the surrounding tissue. No blood means slower nutrient delivery, slower nutrient delivery means slower growth and repair. Ultimately, cartilage damage can necessitate surgical intervention and the need for transplantation, implantation and scaffolding. Given these procedures, it's probably better to hold your nose and swallow the Cod Liver Oil.

There are three types of cartilage: elastic, fibrocartilage and hyaline. Hyaline cartilage is low-friction and found between the joints. Elastic cartilage is the rubbery structure of the ear. Fibrocartilage is tough and found in the knee.

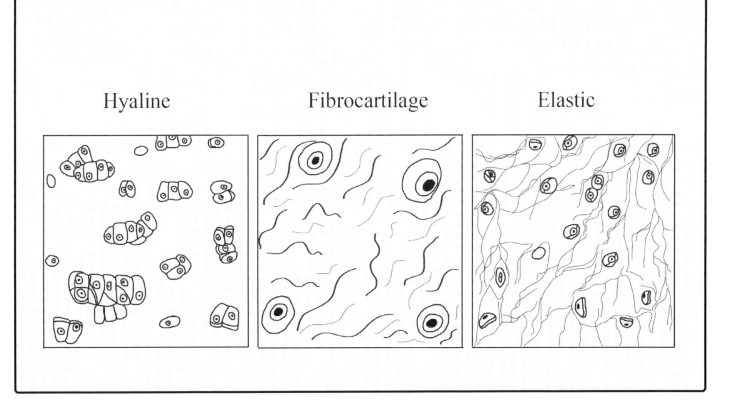

| Hyaline | Fibrocartilage | Elastic |

Notes

_____

Color Key:

HYALINE CARTILAGE
ELASTIC CARTILAGE
FIBROCARTILAGE

CHONDROCYTE, LACUNA, MATRIX,
COLLAGEN FIBER, ELASTIC FIBER

CARTILAGE

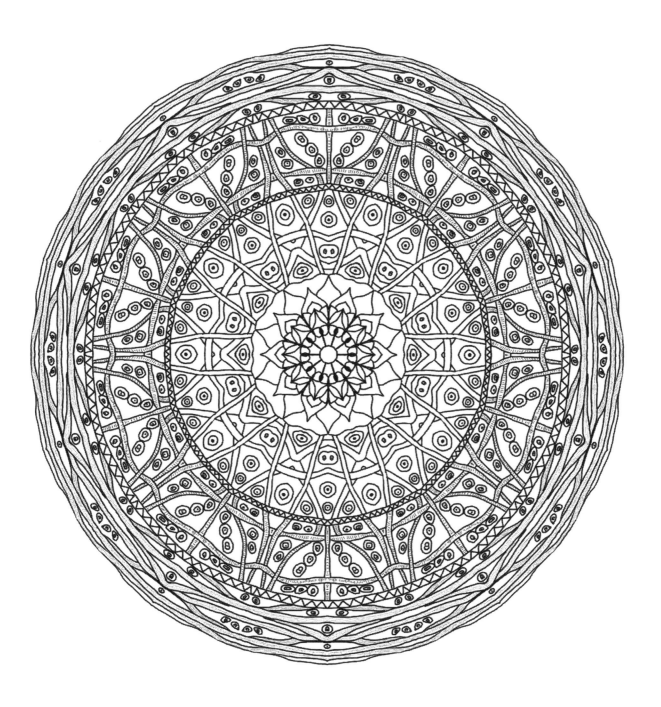

The Pelvis

"Whoever had designed the skeletons of creatures had even less imagination than who designed the outsides. At least the outside-designer had tried a few noveltiesin the spots, wool and stripes department, but the bone-builder had generally just put a skull on a ribcage, shoved a pelvis further along, stuck on some arms and legsand had the rest of the day off. Some ribcages were longer, some legs were shorter, some hands became wings, but they all seemed to be based on one design."

Terry Pratchett, The Last Continent, 1998

The female pelvis and the male pelvis are markedly different, a fact accounted for by the requirements of childbirth. Human infant heads are large and need a wide birth canal if they are to emerge safely from the womb. To accommodate this the female pelvis is broader and shallower, the sciatic notch wider, the pubic symphysis short and the coccyx moveable. These wonders enable childbirth - though the adaptation is far from perfect and the whole process remains painful and risky. For men, the absence of these features means they have narrower hips, and the upshot of that is that men are more efficiently adapted for running as their muscles are more aligned.

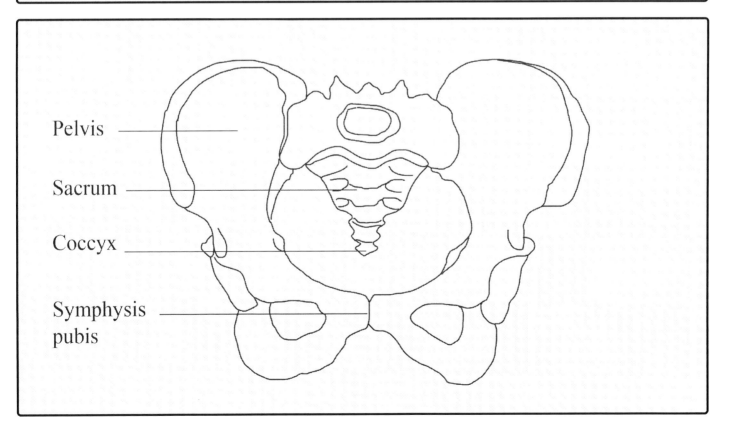

Pelvis

Sacrum

Coccyx

Symphysis
pubis

Notes

_____
_____
_____
_____
_____
_____
_____
_____
_____
_____
_____
_____
_____
_____
_____
_____
_____
_____
_____
_____
_____
_____

Color Key:

WING OF ILIUM
SACRUM
COCCYX
ISCHIUM
PUBIC SYMPHYSIS
PUBIS

PELVIC GIRDLE

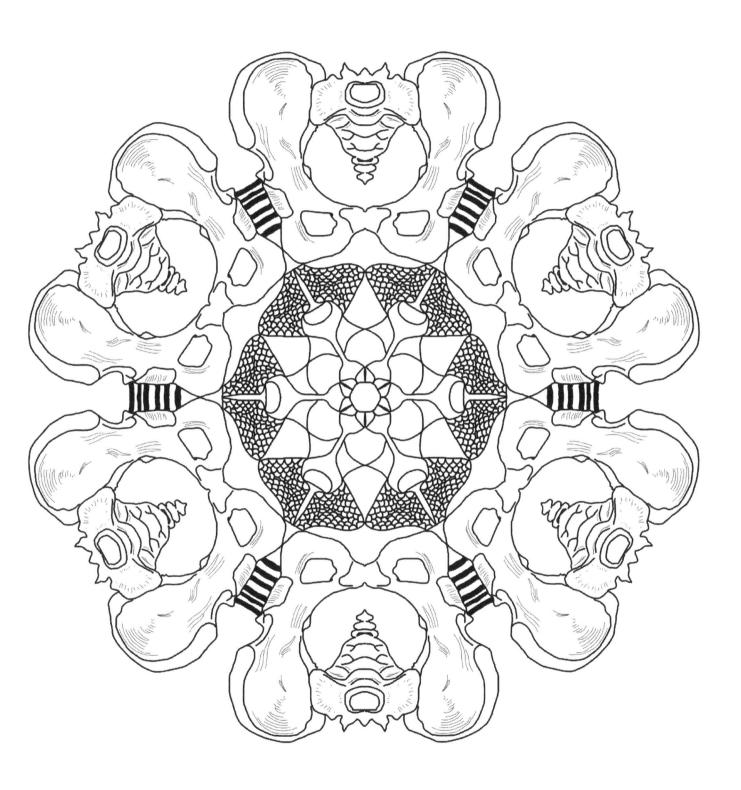

Upper Limbs

"Two little patches of tissue essentially control the development of the pattern of the bones inside limbs. A strip of tissue at the extreme end of the limb bud is essentail for all limb development. Remove it, and development stops. remove it early, and we are left with only an upper arm, or a piece of an arm. remove it slightly later, and we end up with an upper arm and a forearm. remove it even later, and the arm is almost complete, except that the digits are short and deformed."

Neil Shubin, Your Inner Fish: A Journey into the 3.5 Billion Year History of the Human Body, 2008

The skeleton of all mammals have their foundation in a pentadactyl adaptation where the exact form of the upper limb is dependent on the evolved function. "Lucy," the earliest human of the Australopithecus afarensis, has relatively long upper limbs, short lower limbs and a funnel shaped torso. As the need to climb and move through trees dimished over time so too did the length of the human upper limb.

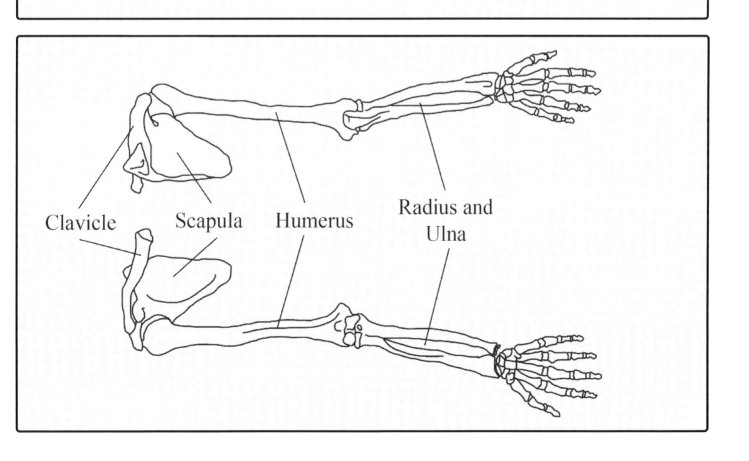

Clavicle   Scapula   Humerus   Radius and Ulna

<u>Notes</u>

Color Key:

CLAVICLE
SCAPULA
HUMERUS
RADIUS
ULNA

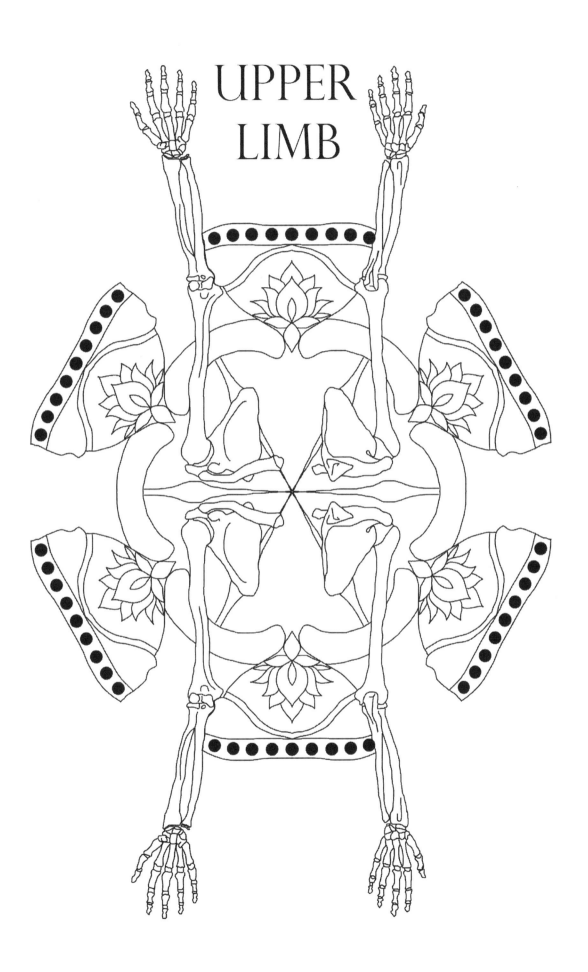

UPPER
LIMB

Tarsals, metatarsals and phalanges

I want to see you
Know your voice
Recognise you when you first come round the corner
Sense your scent when I come
into a room you've just left.
Know the lift of your heel
the glide of your foot
Become familiar with the way
you purse your lips
then let them part
just the slightest bit,
when I lean in to your space
and kiss you
I want to know the joy of how you whisper
"more."

Rumi

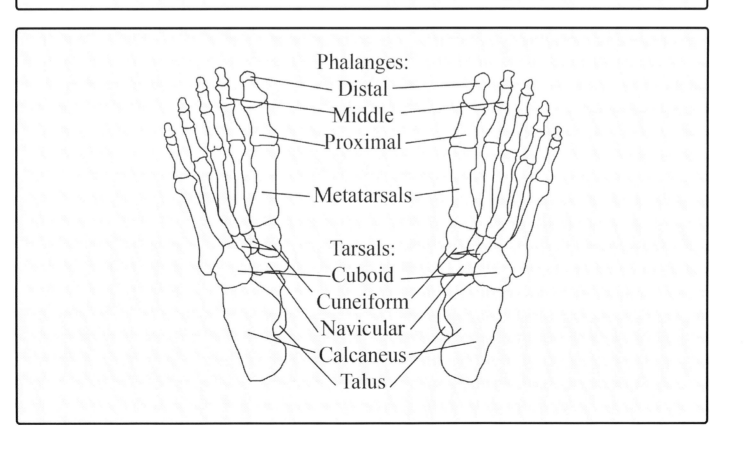

Phalanges:
Distal
Middle
Proximal

Metatarsals

Tarsals:
Cuboid
Cuneiform
Navicular
Calcaneus
Talus

<u>Notes</u>

Color Key:

TARSALS: CALCANEUS, CUBOID, NAVICULAR, CUNEIFORMS

METATARSALS

PHALANGES

Tarsals,Metatarsals & Phalanges

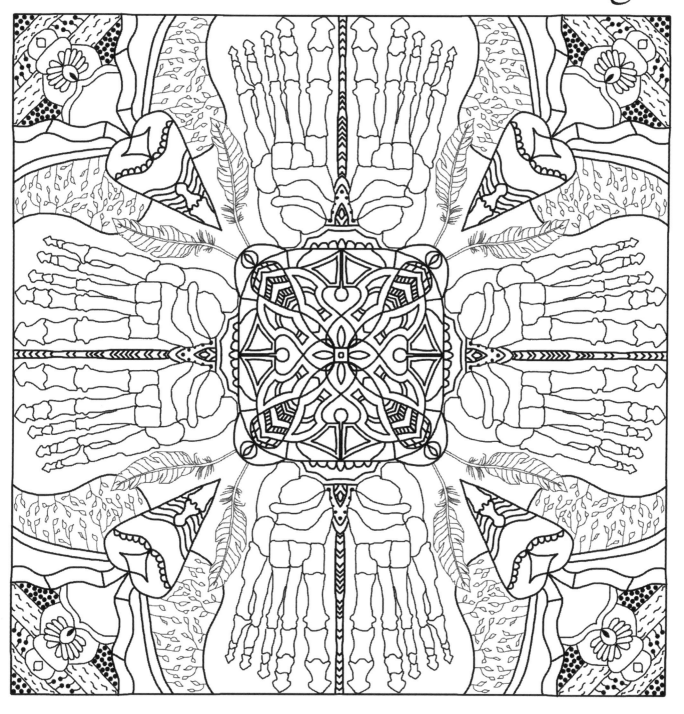

Carpels, Metacarpels and Phalanges

"Indeed, very few people are aware that in each of our fingers, located somewhere between the first phalange, the mesophalange and the metaphalange, there is a tiny brain."

Jose Saramago, The Cave, 2000

Absurd as it sounds, the notion of there being a brain in the hand is an inspired way for accounting for the tactile skill of the artisan craftsman. The dexterity of the fingers, their ability to flex and bend and wiggle is the result of the 27 bones, 27 joints, 34 muscles and over 100 tendons and ligaments. All those distinct parts enable the hands of Saramago's protagonist to glide over the wet slip when fashioning from clay a new piece of pottery. The power grip and the precision grip of the hand enables him to first lift the heavy bags of clay and then, with utmost care, manipulate the tools he uses to create patterns and detailing. The fingers of a single hand are bent and stretched about 25 million times during a single lifetime. And with 17,000 nerve receptors, they are central to our sense of the world.

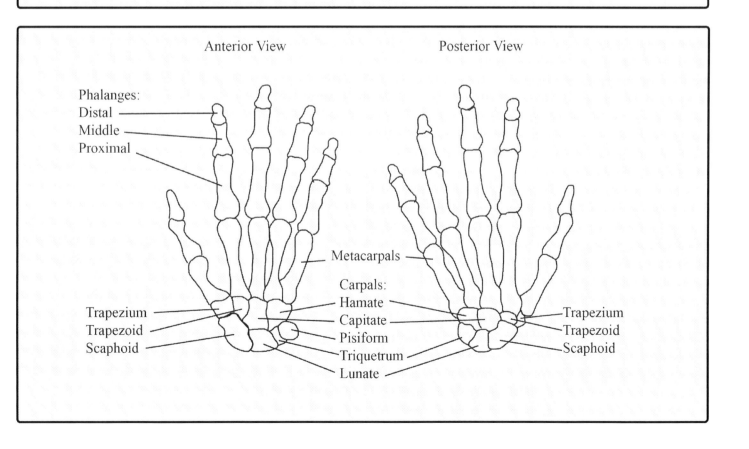

<u>Notes</u>

Color Key:

CARPALS: SCAPHOID, LUNATE,
TRIQUETRUM, PISIFORM,
TRAPEZIUM, TRAPEZOID,
CAPITATE, HAMATE

METACARPALS
PHALANGES.

Carpals, metacarpals and phalanges

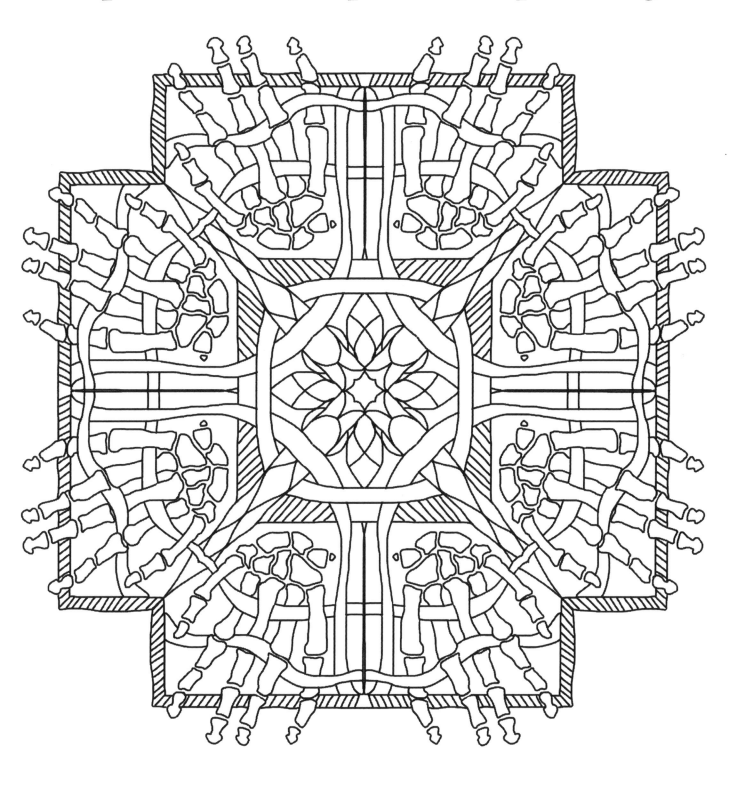

The Skull

"The mind is not a book, to be opened at will and examined at leisure. Thoughts are not etched on the inside of skulls, to be perused by an invader. The mind is a complex and many layered thing, Potter... or at least, most minds are..."

J. K. Rowling, Harry Potter and the Order of the Phoenix, 2003

The human skull can be considered to be formed from three parts: the neurocranium, the sutures and the facial skeleton. There are generally thought to be twenty-two bones within the whole structure, eight forming the brain case and fourteen contributing to the face. That the skull contains and protects the brain is well understood, however, less well known is the long enduring practice of trepanning, which archeological records suggest was performed from the neolithic era onwards. This cross-cultural practice of drilling or scraping a hole into the skull of a person whose behaviour appeared confused or abnormal was seen as a way to release the evil spirits from the heads. As odd as it may seem, this practice endures today in the performance of craniotomy.

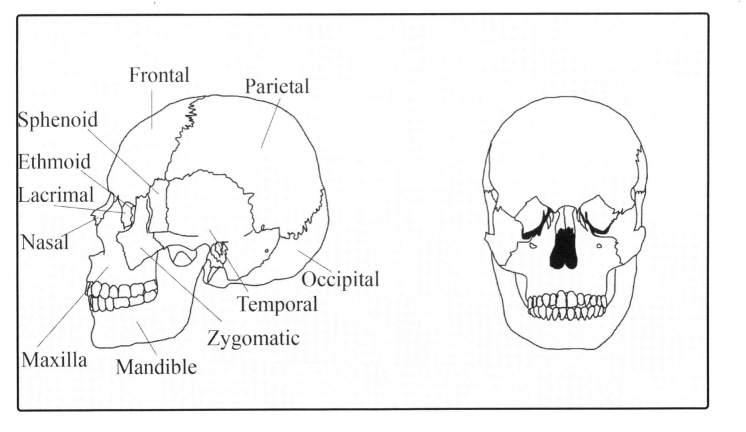

Notes

_____

Color Key:

FRONTAL ; PARIETAL; SPHENOID;
ETHMOID; LACRIMAL; NASAL;
MAXILLA; MANDIBLE; ZYGOMATIC;
TEMPORAL; OCCIPITAL.

THE SKULL

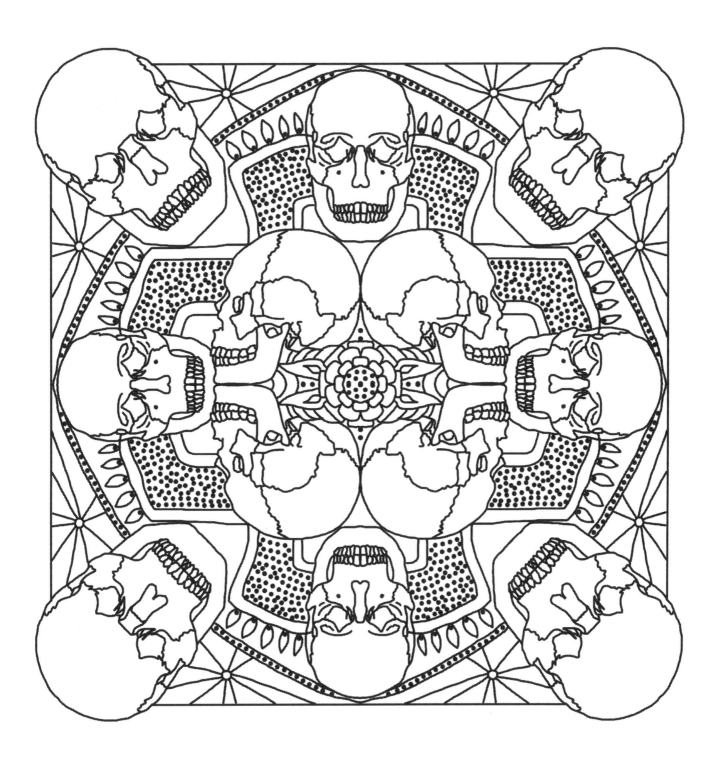

The Heart

"It's really a wonder I haven't dropped all my ideals, because they seem so absurd and impossible to carry out. Yet I keep them, because in spite of everything, I still believe that people are really good at heart."

Anne Frank, The Diary of a Young Girl, 1947

Over the course of a lifetime your heart will beat somewhere in the region of 2.5 billion times. Not once will you need to will it to do so, so faithful will its rhythmic pulse be. The cardiac cycle of coordinated contractions and relaxations causes blood to flow from the atria to the ventricles and so on to the arteries that carry the blood throughout the body. By week five of a pregnancy, two tubes that will become your heart will have formed. Two weeks later the heart will have twisted into a "S" shape and by week nine the four chambers of the heart will have formed. Because the lungs of a baby are filled with a fluid until birth and so do not supply oxygen, the wall between the two atria of a foetus's heart has a small opening, the fossa ovalis. In most cases, it closes within a few months after birth. However, it remains true to say that before we were born we all had a small hole in our heart.

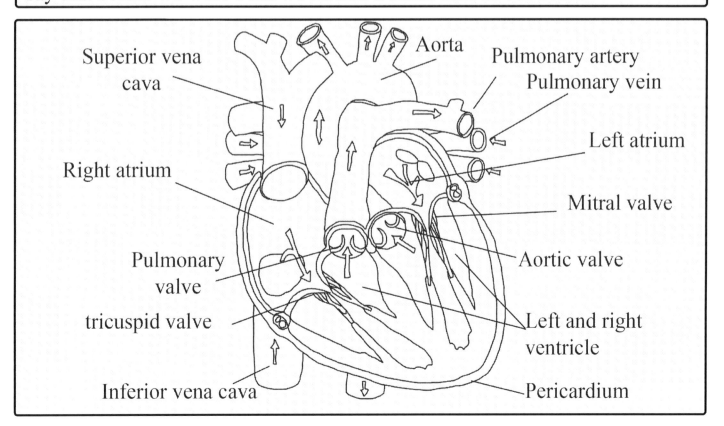

Notes

Color Key:

AORTA
PULMONARY ARTERY
ATRIA
VENTRICLE
TRICUSPID VALVE
AORTIC VALVE
MITRAL VALVE

THE HEART

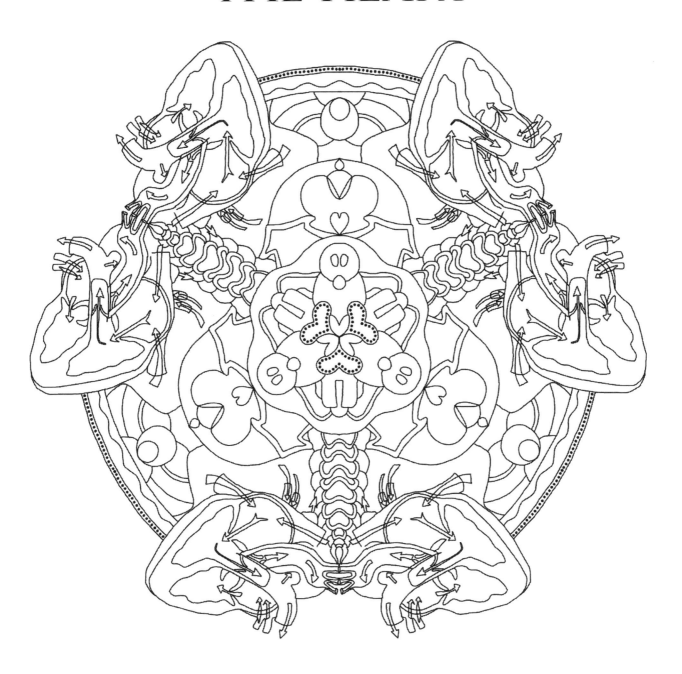

The Lungs

I felt my lungs inflate with the onrush of scenery - air, mountains, trees, people. I thought, "This is what it is to be happy."

Sylvia Plath, The Bell Jar, 1963

The respiratory tract extends from the nostrils to the alveoli of the lungs and has the unique function of allowing the exchange of gases between the inside and outside of the body. It is also home to a niche-specific microbiome that serves to protect us from air-borne pathogens. These microbial communities have co-existed with humans for millions of years and have become a major contributor to our overall health. The human airways have a total surface area of approximately 70 m^2, which is roughly 40 times larger than that of the skin. In this regard, it is true to say that the place where we come most into contact with the outside world is within the respiratory tract. Naturally enough, the airways are therefore susceptible to an onslaught of infection and it is the symbiotic relationship between human and microbiota that occurs in the mucosa of the trachea that helps to guard against disease.

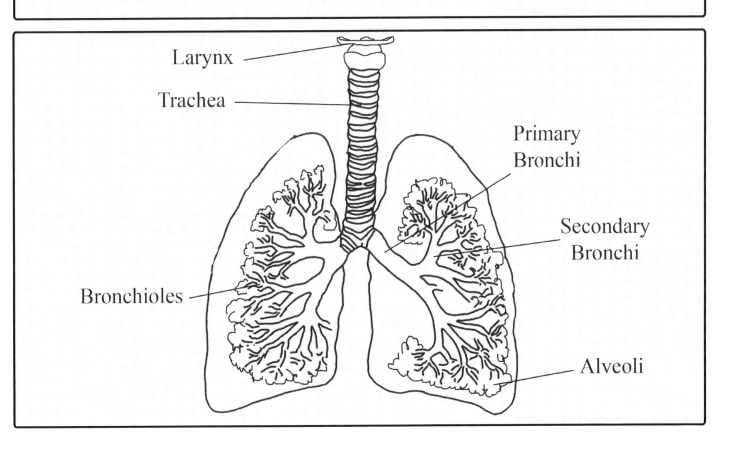

<u>Notes</u>

Color Key:

LARYNX
TRACHEA
PRIMARY BRONCHI
SECONDARY BRONCHI
BRONCHIOLES
ALVEOLI

THE LUNGS

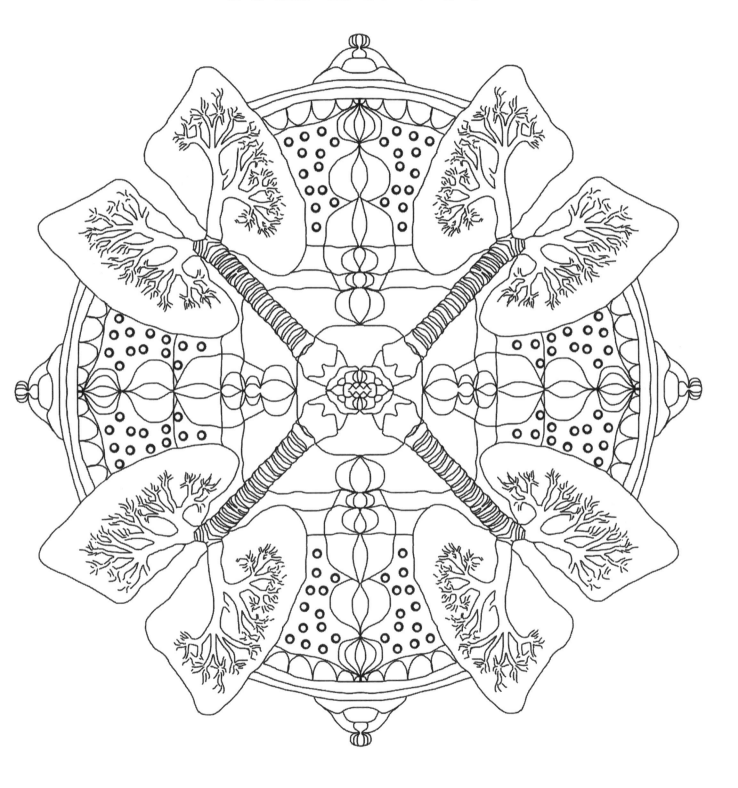

Respiratory System

"Influenza is not simply a bad cold. It is a quite specific disease, with a distinct set of symptoms and epidemiological behaviour. In humans the virus directly attacks the respiratory system, and it becomes increasingly dangerous as it penetrates deeper into the lungs. Indirectly it affects many parts of the body, and even a mild infection can cause pain in muscles and joints, intense headache, and prostration."

John M Barry, The Great Influenza, 2004

The respiratory system delivers to the body the oxygen that is needed for life. Relying on a concentration gradient between the gases carried in the blood and the gases in the alveoli, respiration occurs because oxygen and carbon dioxide can diffuse across the the capillary walls. The air enters the alveoli when the diagphram causes a change in pressure that inflates the lungs. A simple enough autonomic process, but one that is essential for human life. Live to the ripe age of 80 years and you will have taken 672 million breaths, breathed in some of the same atoms as Leonardo da Vinci and exhaled about one cup of water for every day you lived.

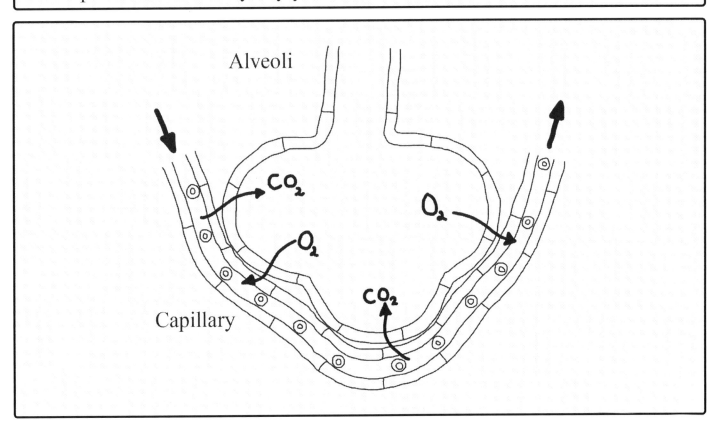

Notes

Respiratory System

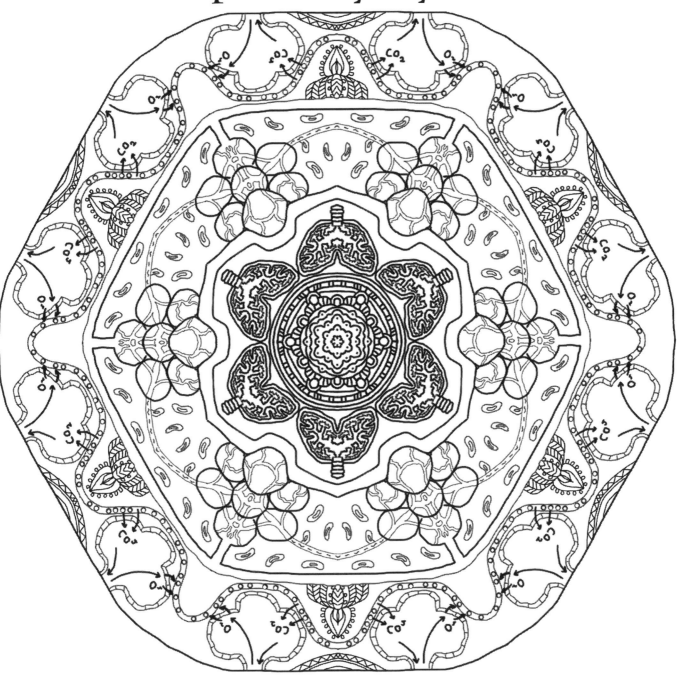

Abdominal Organs

"The abdomen is the reason why man does not easily take himself for a god."
Friedrich Nietzsche, Beyond Good and evil, 1886

Rammed with the vital organs of the body, the abdomen is understandably a place of concern for medics. Gastrointestinal disease is one of the most frequently cited causes of sudden natural death, and the range of diseases and disorders found within this region of the body is legion. From peptic ulcers to gastroparesis, cirrhosis to hepatitis, diabetes to pancreatitis, Whipple's disease to inflammatory bowel disease, and Crohn's disease to colon cancer, the abdominal organs can be a source of great suffering and medical intrigue. And yet, the viscera are fundamental to our digestive system, which means they are deliciously proximal to our enjoyment of food. Every morsel finds its final bodily destination in the rectum of the colon, having passed through the stomach and intestines where the nutrients and goodness have been extracted. Eat well and your abdomen will thank you, indulge in the worst of foods and you could well pay with your life.

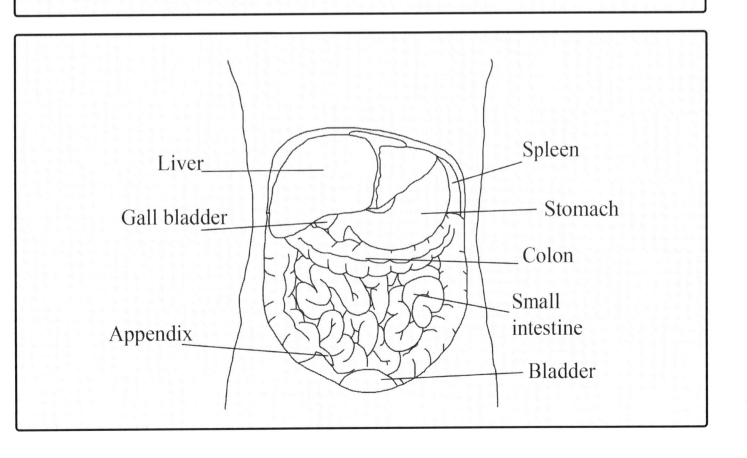

Liver

Gall bladder

Appendix

Spleen

Stomach

Colon

Small intestine

Bladder

Notes

_____

ABDOMINAL ORGANS

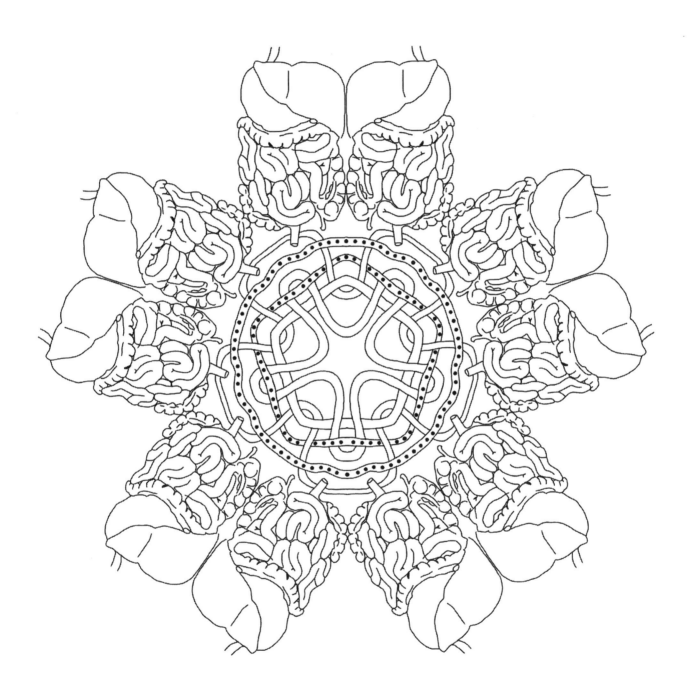

Large Intestine

"The advent of cooking enabled humans to eat more kinds of food, to devote less time to eating, and to make do with smaller teeth and shorter intestines.Some scholars believe there is a direct link between the advent of cooking, the shortening of the intestinal tract, and the growth of the human brain. Since long intestines and large brains are both massive energy consumers, it's hard to have both."

Yuval Noah Harari, Sapiens: A Brief History of Humankind, 2011

The large intestine and its bacterial population do much more than store the waste from our body. Divided into four sections, the caecum, colon, rectum and anal canal, it is about 1.5 m long and has a diameter of approximately 6 cm. Along its length, the large intestine serves to reabsorb water and mineral ions, as well as forming and storing faeces, maintaining a colony of over 500 types of bacteria and providing a place for bacterial fermentation to occur. There is also a network of interconnected nerve cells within the organ that acts as a "second brain" - the emerging field of neurogastroenterology is investigating how the large intestine affects the body's immune defence.

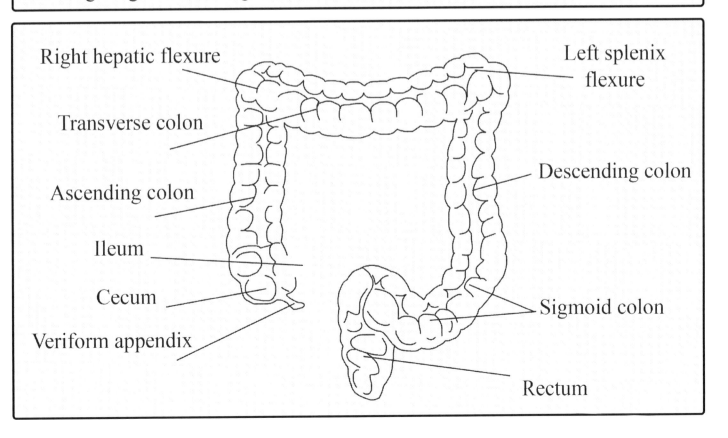

Right hepatic flexure
Left splenix flexure
Transverse colon
Descending colon
Ascending colon
Ileum
Cecum
Sigmoid colon
Veriform appendix
Rectum

<u>Notes</u>

Color Key:

CAECUM
ASCENDING COLON
TRANSVERSE COLON
DESCENDING COLON
SIGNOID COLON
RECTUM

LARGE INTESTINE

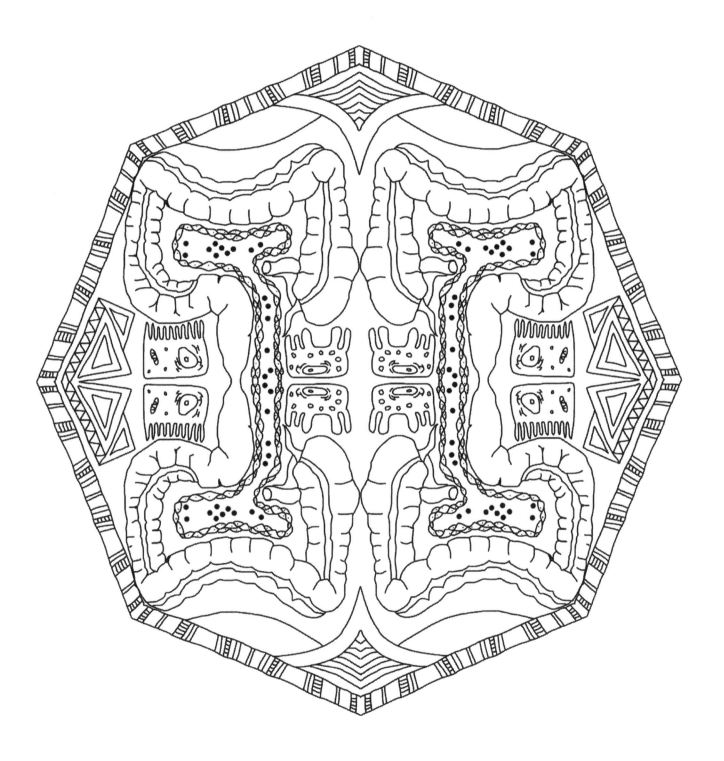

Small Intestine

"When I was small and would leaf through the Old Testament retold for children and illustrated in engravings by Gustave Dore, I saw the Lord God standing on a cloud. He was an old man with eyes, nose and a long beard, and I would say to myself that if He had a mouth, He had to eat. And if He ate, He had intestines. But that always gave me a fright, because even though I come from a family that was not particularly religious, I felt the idea of a divine intestine to be sacriligious."

Milan Kundera, The Unbearable Lightness of Being, 1984

What makes the thought of a divine intestine so unthinkble for Kundera's protagonist must relate to the function of the organ. If the problem of evil is not disturbing, why should the intestine be so abject? In breaking down food from the stomach and absorbing the nutrients therein, the small intestines serve to process the food we eat into something the body can incorporate. However, for Kundera, the problem arises as the aftermath of this process - the idea of waste and excrement. God, by virtue of having a mouth, and therefore an intestine that can process the food, is responsible for excrement also.

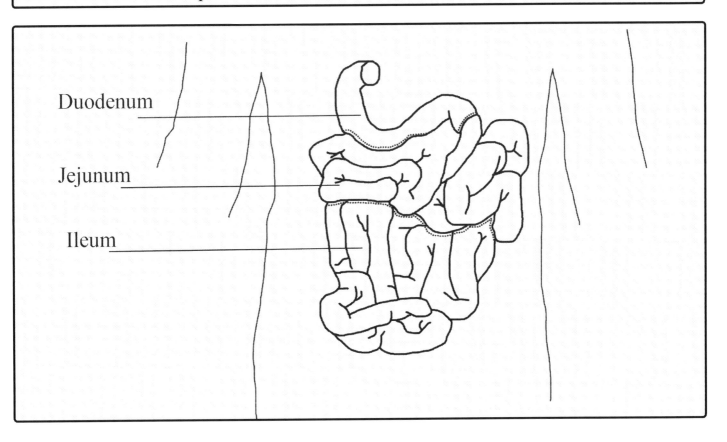

Duodenum

Jejunum

Ileum

Notes

_____
_____
_____
_____
_____
_____
_____
_____
_____
_____
_____
_____
_____
_____
_____
_____
_____
_____
_____
_____
_____

Color Key:

DUODENUM
JEJUNUM
ILEUM

VILLI
EPTHELIAL CELLS (WITH MICRO VILLI)

THE SMALL INTESTINE

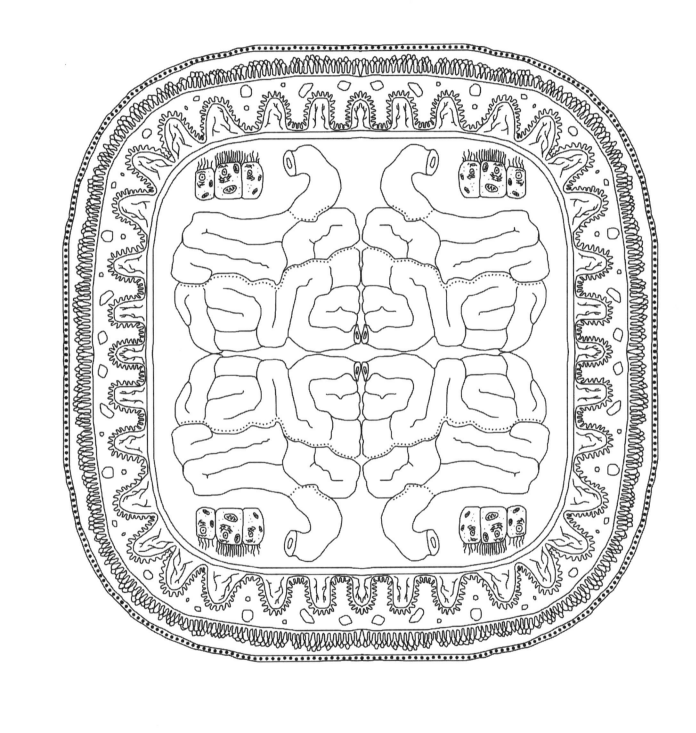

The Liver

"May I urge you to consider my liver?" asked the animal, "it must be very rich and tender by now, I've been force feeding myself for months."
Douglas Adams, The Restaurant at the End of the Universe, 1980

The largest solid organ in the body, the liver has the role of detoxifying the blood, manufacturing proteins and hormones, and fighting infection. In fact, and rather astonishingly, the liver has over 500 other jobs all aimed at maintaining the balance of one's health. Unique amongst human organs, and much like a lizard's tail, the liver has the capacity to regenerate itself, so that when a portion is transplanted, the donor's liver will grow back to its original size and the recipient's portion will attain the size required by the new body.

However, force feeding ducks and geese and causing their livers to swell up to ten times their usual size, causing hepatic lipidosis and other diseases, causing bacterial and fungal infections, is no way to produce a luxury food item to the highest of animal welfare standards.

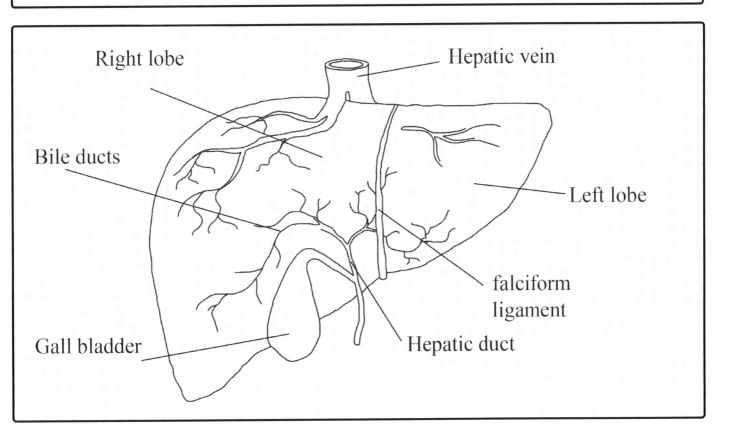

Notes

Color Key:

TERMINAL BRANCH OF HEPATIC VEIN
BILE DUCT
PORTAL VEIN
HEPATIC ARTERY
HEPATOCYTE

STRUCTURE OF THE LIVER

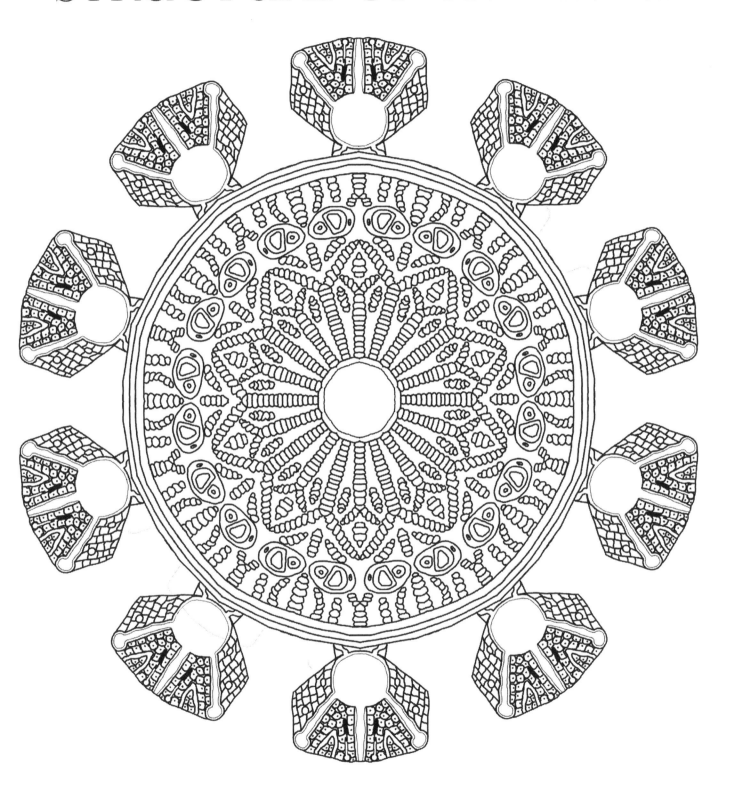

The Pancreas

"When blood-sugar (glucose) levels rise, the pancreas secretes insulin in response, which then signals the muscles to take up and burn more glucose. Insulin also signals the cells to take up fat and hold on to it. Only when the rising tide of blood sugar begins to ebb will insulin levels ebb as well, at which point the fat cells will release their stored fuel into circulation (in the form of fatty acids); the cells of muscles and organs now burn this fat rather than gluscose."

Gary Taubes, The Case Against Sugar, 2016

And there you have it. The pancreas has two functions: an exocrine function that helps to digest food and an endocrine function that regulates blood sugar. By producing insulin, which acts to lower blood sugar, and glucagon, which acts to raise it, the pancreas works hard to maintain the proper blood-sugar levels required by the brain, liver and kidneys.

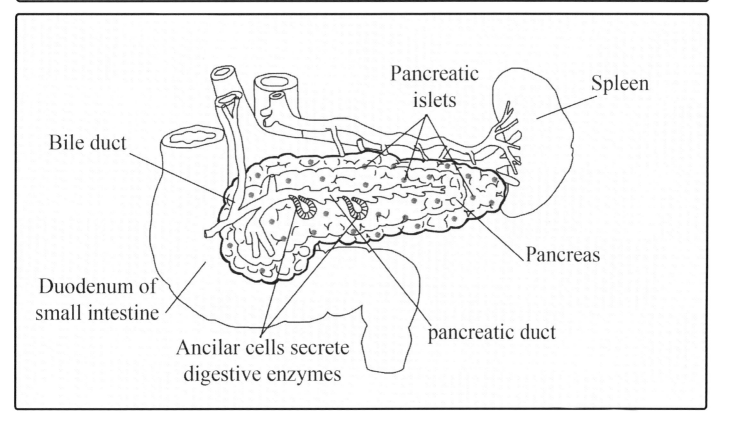

Pancreatic islets

Spleen

Bile duct

Pancreas

Duodenum of small intestine

pancreatic duct

Ancilar cells secrete digestive enzymes

Notes

Color Key:

PANCREATIC DUCT
DIGESTIVE ENZYME SECRETING CELL
ISLET OF LANGERHANS
CAPILLARY
HORMONE SECTRING ISLET CELL

ANATOMY OF THE PANCREAS

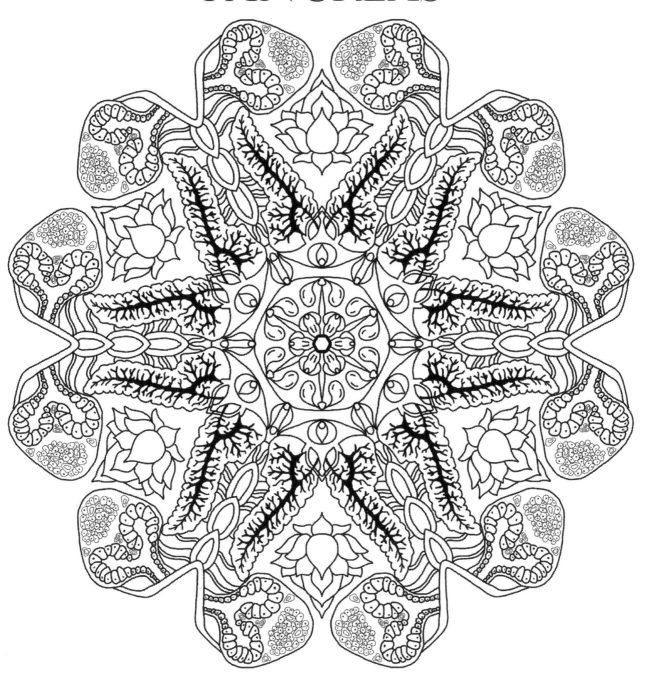

Kidney

"Mr Leopold Bloom ate with relish the inner organs of beasts and fowls. He liked thick giblet soup, nutty gizzards, a stuffed roast heart, liverslices fried with crustcrumbs, fried hencods' roes. Most of all he liked grilled mutton kidneys, which gave to his palate a fine tang of faintly scented urine."

James Joyce, Ulysses, 1922

Joyce's characterisation of the kidney is a little unfair. As humorous as it may be to cast the kidney as a urine factory, this fist-sized organ is no one-trick pony. Not only does the kidney remove waste products and drugs from the body, it also helps to balance the body fluids, releases hormones that regulate blood pressure, produces vitamin D to promote strong healthy bones, and controls the production of red blood cells. Each kidney, you have two on either side of the lowest part of the ribcage, contains about a million functioning units called nephrons. These nephrons filter the blood and the waste material is added to water and a mix of chemicals to produce urine.

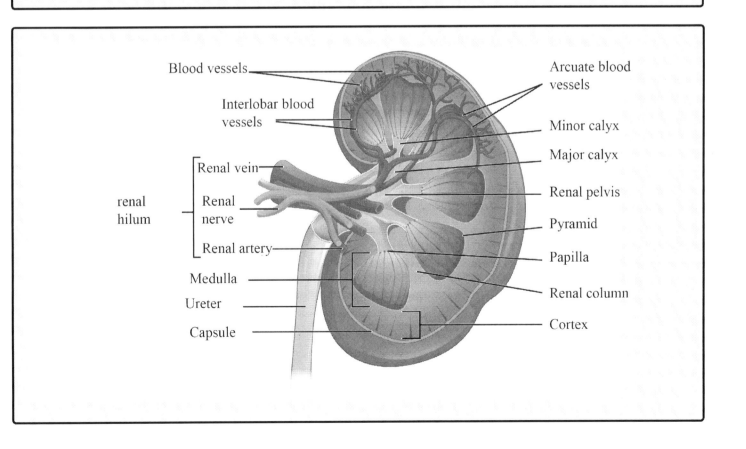

<u>Notes</u>

Color Key:

RENAL ARTERY
RENAL VEIN
AORTA
URETER
MEDULLA
CORTEX
RENAL PYRAMID

ANATOMY OF THE KIDNEY

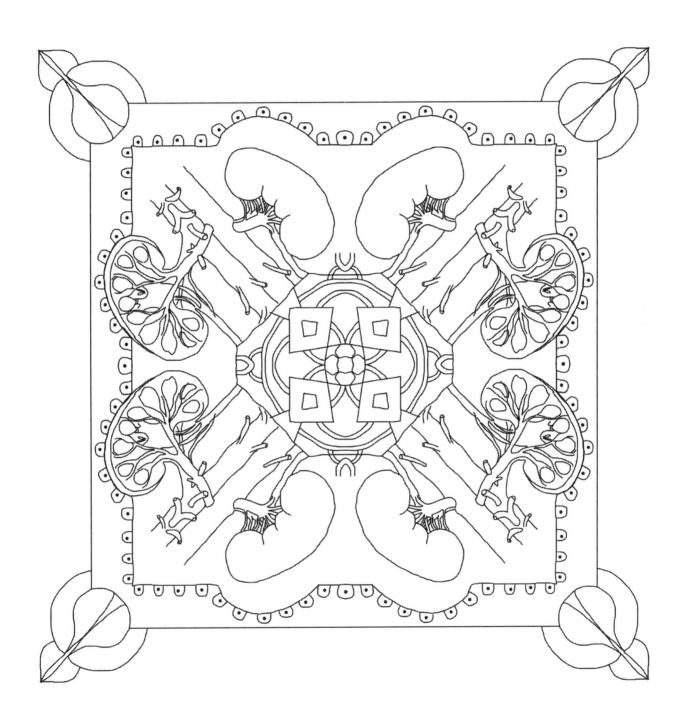

Neurons

"The human brain, it has to be said, is the most complexly organised structure in the entire universe and to appreciate this you just have to look at some numbers. The brain is made up of one hundred billion nerve cells or "neurons," which are the basic structural and functional units of the nervous system. Each neuron makes something like a thousand to ten thousand contacts with other neurons and these points of contact are called synapses, where exchange of information occurs. And based on this information, someone has calculated that the number of possible permutations and combinations of brain activity, in other words the number of brain states, exceeds the number of elementary particles in the known universe."

V. S. Ramachandran, Reith lecture, 2003

And if this wasn't incredible enough, new neurons are made in just two parts of the brain - the hippocampus and the olfactory bulb - all the others are the same age as you, they've celebrated every birthday you've ever had and will be with you until your dying day. They don't divide and may even outlast the body that contains them.

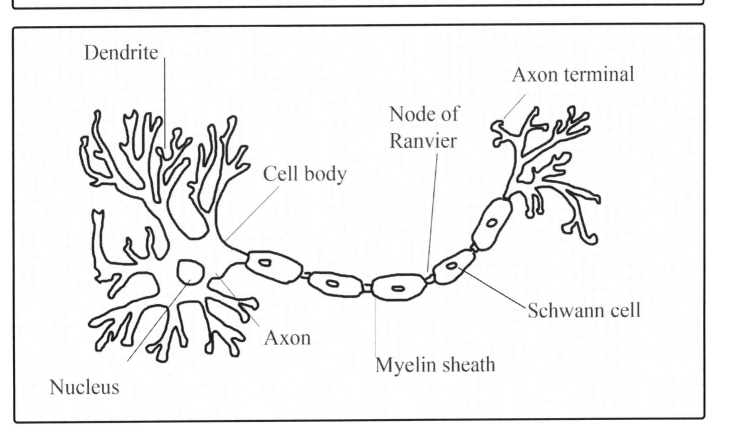

<u>Notes</u>

Color Key:

AXON TERMINAL
SCHWANN CELL
MYELIN SHEATH
AXON
NUCLEUS
CELL BODY
DENDRITE

Neuron

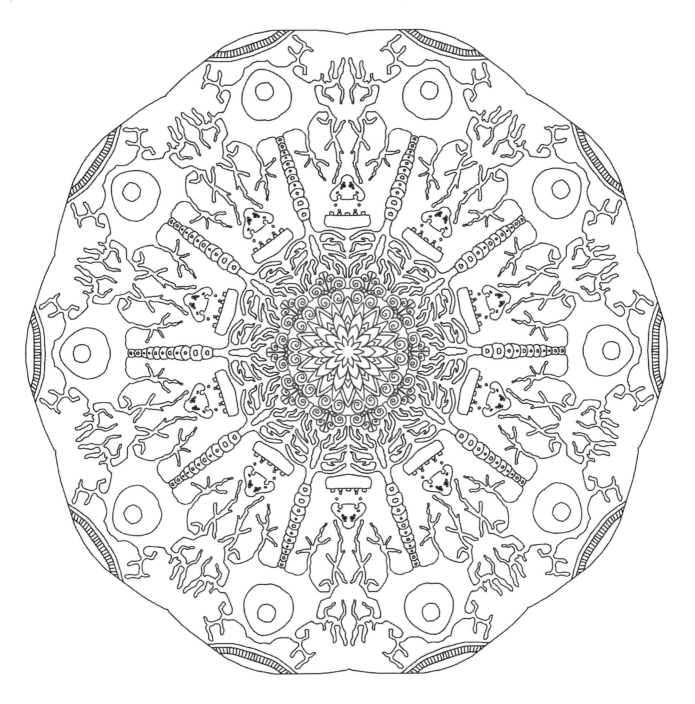

The Brain

"Finally, from so little sleeping and so much reading, his brain dried up and he went completely out of his mind."

Miguel de Cervantes, Don Quixote, 1605

The most complex organ in the body, the brain is the locus of the ultimate mystery - consciousness and our sense of being. Poke around in the brain and you might learn how the brain processes and stores information, how neuroplasticity allows for learning throughout the course of one's life, and how language and the ability to determine meaning develop during childhood. Yet, despite all that we have learnt, there remains a central philosophical conundrum when we try to understand subjective experience through objective means. The cerebral cortex has been identified as a region of importance for consciousness since the nineteenth century, however it has become increasingly obvious that there is not one single location for consciousness. Our awarenes of the world, and of our selfhood in the world, is spread across the whole of the brain, with studies of conscious and unconscious patients providing evidence of how complex the situation remains.

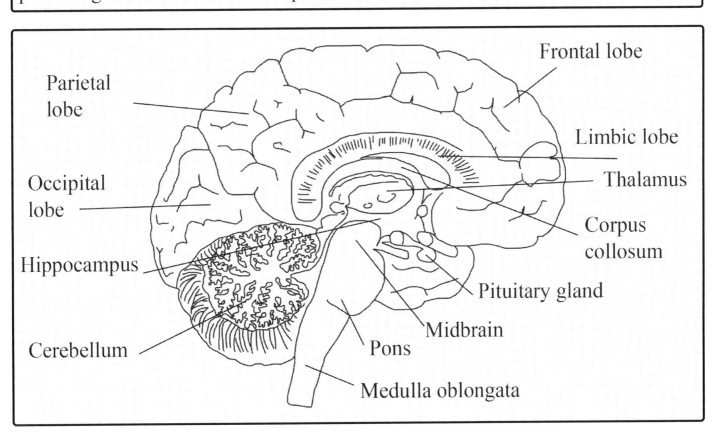

<u>Notes</u>

Color Key:

THE BRAIN

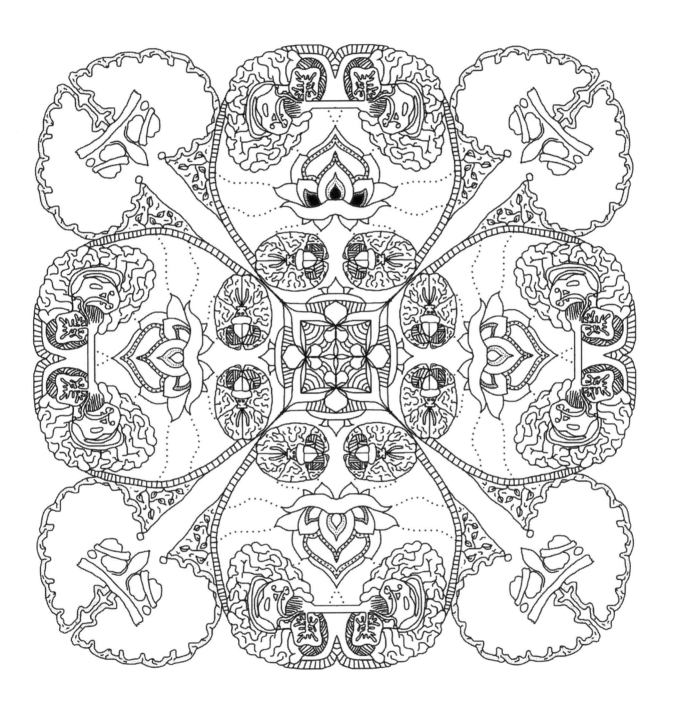

Cranial Nerves

"A branch of one of the cranial nerves, the recurrent laryngeal, runs from the brain to the larynx. It doesn't go straight there, however. Instead, it dives down to the chest, loops around one of the main arteries leaving the heart, and proceeds back up the neck to the larynx. In a giraffe the detour is significant (British understatement) and it is presumably costly. The explanation lies in history, in the nerve's emergence in our fish ancestors before a discernible neck evolved."

Richard Dawkins, Brief Candle in the Dark: My Life in Science, 2015

Cranial nerves act as either one-way or two-way communication channels for the brain. Those that transmit information to the brain are termed afferent (Nerves I, II and VIII), while those that transmit instructions from the brain are efferent (Nerves III, IV, VI, XI, and XII). The remaining nerves (V, VII, IX and X) function to carry information in both directions. Ten of the twelve cranial nerves originate in the braistem, which connects the cerebrum and cerebellum to the spinal cord.

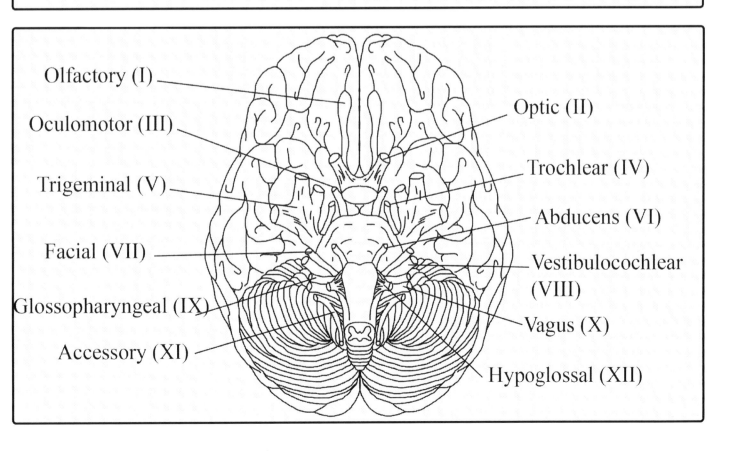

Olfactory (I)
Oculomotor (III)
Trigeminal (V)
Facial (VII)
Glossopharyngeal (IX)
Accessory (XI)
Optic (II)
Trochlear (IV)
Abducens (VI)
Vestibulocochlear (VIII)
Vagus (X)
Hypoglossal (XII)

Notes

TWELVE CRANIAL NERVES

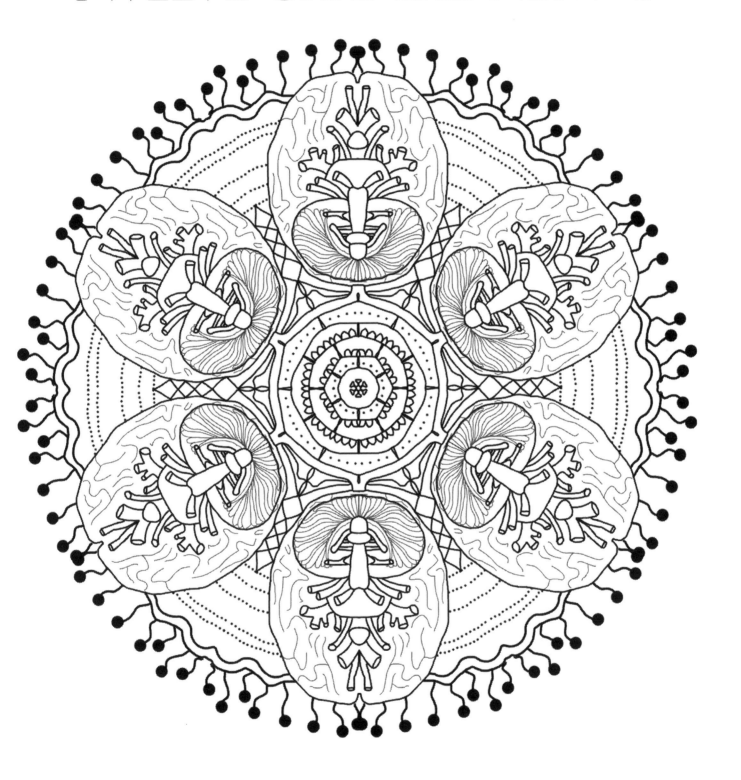

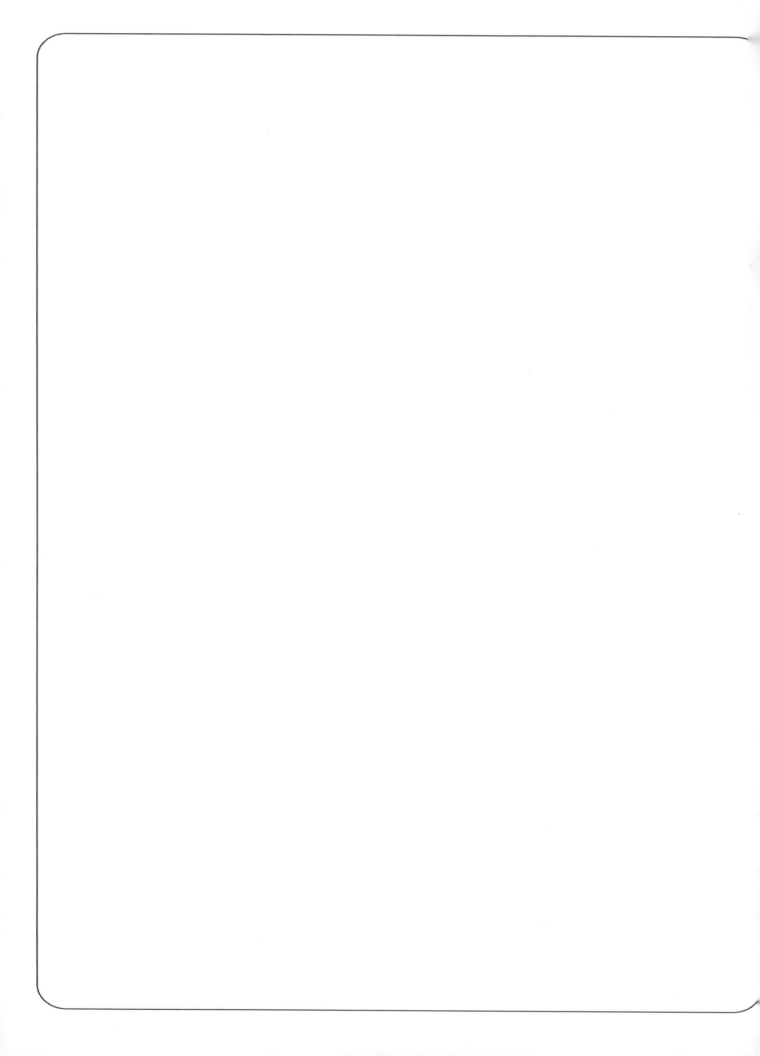

Spinal Column and Cord

"If someone can enjoy marching to music in rank and file, I can feel only contempt for him; he has received his large brain by mistake, a spinal cord would have been enough."

Albert Einstein, The World as I See It, 1934

The spinal cord is the vital bridge between the brain and the body. Running 40 - 50 cm down through the spinal column, the spinal cord has 31 pairs of nerves emerging from the white and grey matter of its four regions: cervical, thoracic, lumbar and sacral. These nerves carry sensory information from the body to the central nervous system, though the spinal cord also performs the initial processing of these sensations as well as mediating the autonomic control of most of the visceral functions. Severing the cord effectively separates the brain from the rest of the body, which makes it of immense clinical significance. It is rare that it is completely severed, however. A chest (thoracic) or lower back (lumbar) injury might affect the functioning of your legs, torso, bowels and sexual organs, while a neck (cervical) injury would likely also affect movement in one's arms and possibly one's breathing.

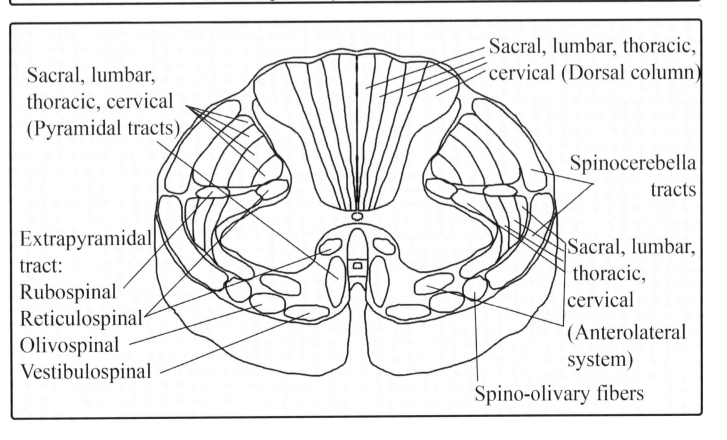

Sacral, lumbar, thoracic, cervical (Dorsal column)

Sacral, lumbar, thoracic, cervical (Pyramidal tracts)

Spinocerebella tracts

Extrapyramidal tract:
Rubospinal
Reticulospinal
Olivospinal
Vestibulospinal

Sacral, lumbar, thoracic, cervical (Anterolateral system)

Spino-olivary fibers

Notes

SPINAL COLUMN AND CORD

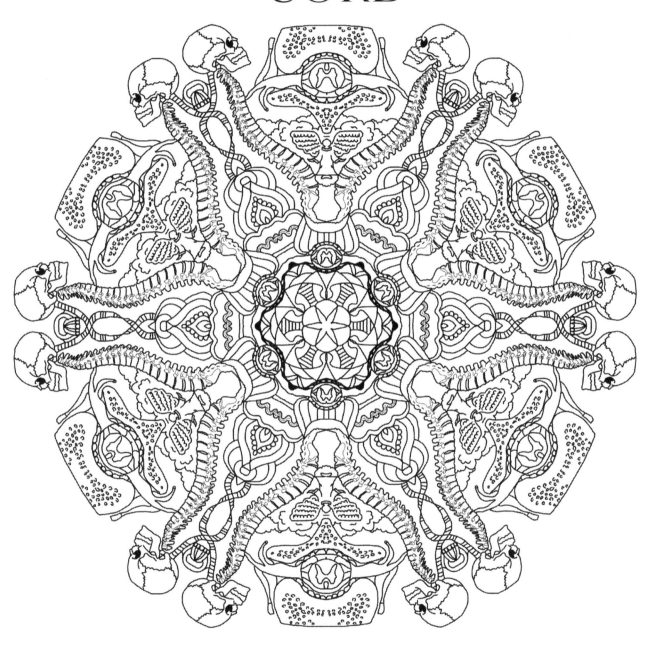

Synapse

"Science finds it difficult to decipher the mysteries of the mind largely because we lack efficient tools. Many people, including many scientists, tend to confuse the mind with the brain, but they are really very different things. The brain is a material network of neurons, synapses and biochemicals. The mind is a flow of subjective experiences, such as pleasure, pain, anger and love. Biologists assume that the brain somehow produces the mind, and that biochemical reactions in billions of neurons somehow produce experiences such as pain and love. However, so far we have absolutely no explanation for how the mind emerges from the brain."

Yuval Noah Harari, 21 Lessons for the 21st Century, 2018

The biochemical reactions that are mentioned in the quote are the millions of interactions that occur in the synaptic cleft between two neurons. Neurotransmitters pass from the axon terminal of one neuron and attach themselves to the receptors of another neuron, a muscle cell or a gland. In doing so, they activate the target cell, which is excited or inhibited according to which of the over 100 neurotransmitters has passed on the message.

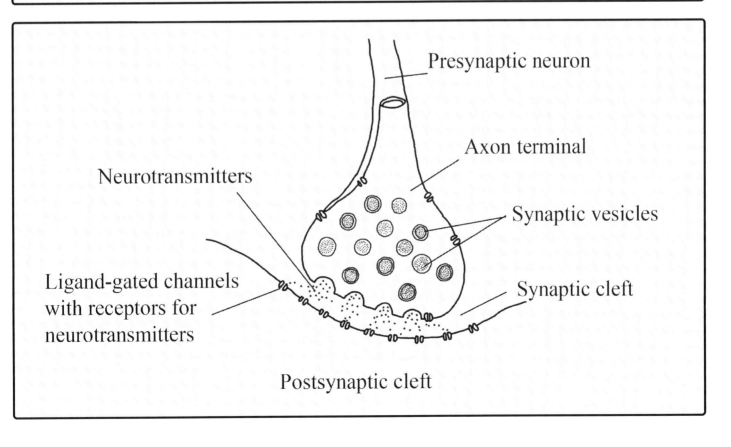

Presynaptic neuron

Axon terminal

Neurotransmitters

Synaptic vesicles

Ligand-gated channels with receptors for neurotransmitters

Synaptic cleft

Postsynaptic cleft

Notes

Color Key:

SYNAPTIC VESICLE
MITOCHONDRIA
NEUROTRANSMITTER
RECEPTOR
ION CHANNEL
CYTOPLASM

Synapses

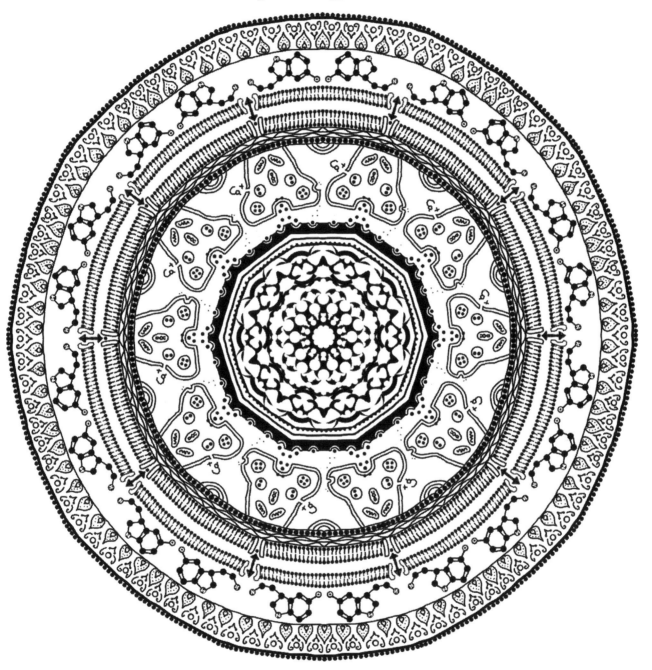

Touch - Integument

"Man is an onion made up of a hundred integuments, a texture made up of many threads. The ancient Asiatics knew this well enough, and in the Buddhist yoga an exact technique was devised for unmasking the illusion of the personality. The human merry-go-round sees many changes: the illusion that cost India the efforts of thousands of years to unmask is the same illusion that the West has labored just as hard to maintain and strengthen."

Hermann Hesse, Steppenwolf, 1927

The skin is an organ that can respond to sensations and send messages to the brain that is then able to decipher the kind of experience felt. Through haptic perception, the skin enables us to detect changes in temperature, pressure, texture and to experience tickly, itchy and painful sensations. The sensory nerve fibers within the dermis form the somatosensory system and conduct an electrical discharge up the spinal cord to the parietal lobe of the brain. The pacinian corpuscles in the dermis respond to forces and record deep-pressure touch and high-frequency vibrations.

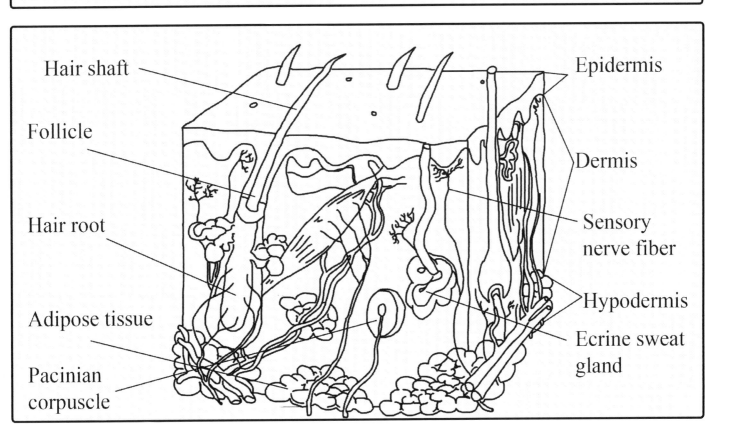

Hair shaft

Follicle

Hair root

Adipose tissue

Pacinian corpuscle

Epidermis

Dermis

Sensory nerve fiber

Hypodermis

Ecrine sweat gland

Notes

_____

_____

_____

_____

_____

_____

_____

_____

_____

_____

_____

_____

_____

_____

_____

_____

_____

_____

_____

_____

Color Key:

EPIDERMIS: CORNEUM, GRANULOSUM, BASALE

DERMIS: NERVE/RECEPTOR, ARTERY/VEIN, LYMPHATIC VESSEL, HAIR FOLLICLE, SEBACEOUS GLAND,

SUPERFICIAL FASCIA

THE INTEGUMENT

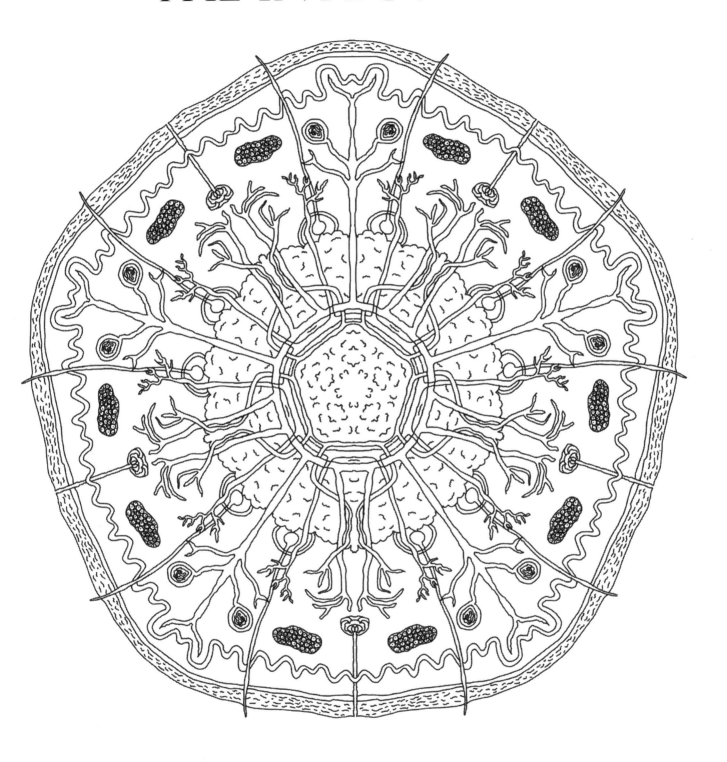

Taste - The Tongue

"Some books should be tasted, some devoured, but only a few should be chewed and digested thoroughly."

Francis Bacon

Our sense of taste is so closely bound to our emotions that it has been incorporated into out metaphoric language. We speak of feeling bitter when something hasn't gone our way, of the sweetness of someone's smile, and of the saltiness of a rebuke. Each of these tastes, along with sourness and umami, have a specific location on the tongue and are processed in particular regions of the brain. Such is the power of these metaphors that simply reading a sentence that utilises taste in this way is enough to elicit brain activity in these regions. The tongue itself is lined by stratified squamous epithelium and houses a field of raised bumps called papilla. These bumps, of which there are three types, contain the taste buds, with each bud being formed from several gustatory receptor cells. Neurotransmitters in these cells are released when certain chemicals are detected, and messages are then sent to the facial and glossopharyngeal cranial nerves.

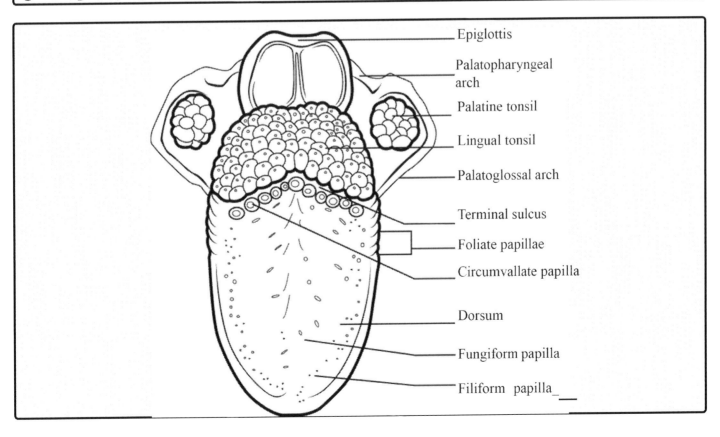

Notes

Color Key:

PAPILLAE: CIRCUM VALLATE, FUNGIFORM, FILIFORM

TASTE BUD: PORE CANAL, RECEPTOR CELL, SUPPORTING CELL, NERVE FIBER

SWEET, SOUR, SALT, BITTER, UMAMI

THE TONGUE

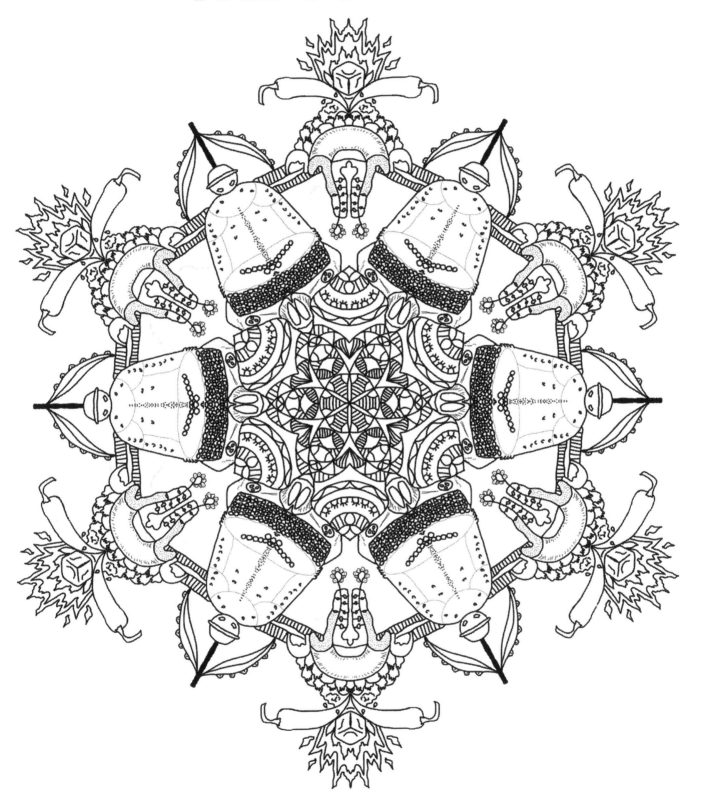

Smell - The Nose

"The human olfactory system is atrophied; roughly forty percent of a rat's brain is devoted to olfactory processing, versus three percent in us."

Robert M Sapolsky, Behave: The Biology of Our Best and Worst, 2017

Recent research has established that the human nose can detect at least one trillion distinct scents. It is able to do this because of the vast number of scent receptors in the olfactory cleft and the myriad permutations in which they can be combined. These cells form the only cranial nerve that can be renewed, regenerating themselves every 30-60 days, a process that has possibly been going on for as long as there has been life on Earth, since even single-celled microorganisms have ways of detecting the chemical environment in which they are immersed. Smell is, after all, the process of chemical detection. And yet it is also closely associated with emotion, so much so that the emotions of fear and disgust produce their own chemical signature. With that in mind, perhaps our thoughts should be with man's best friend - they have over 40 times as many scent receptors as us.

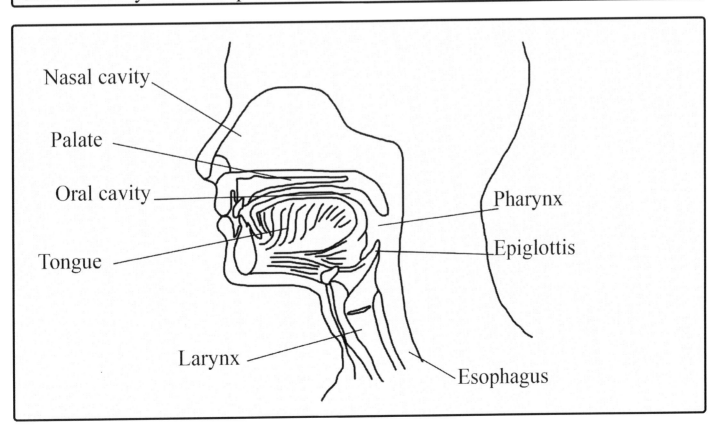

Notes

_____
_____
_____
_____
_____
_____
_____
_____
_____
_____
_____
_____
_____
_____
_____
_____
_____
_____
_____

Color Key:

- NASAL CAVITY
- UVULA
- PHARYNX
- EPIGLOTTIS
- ESOPHAGUS
- LARYNX

THE NASAL CAVITY

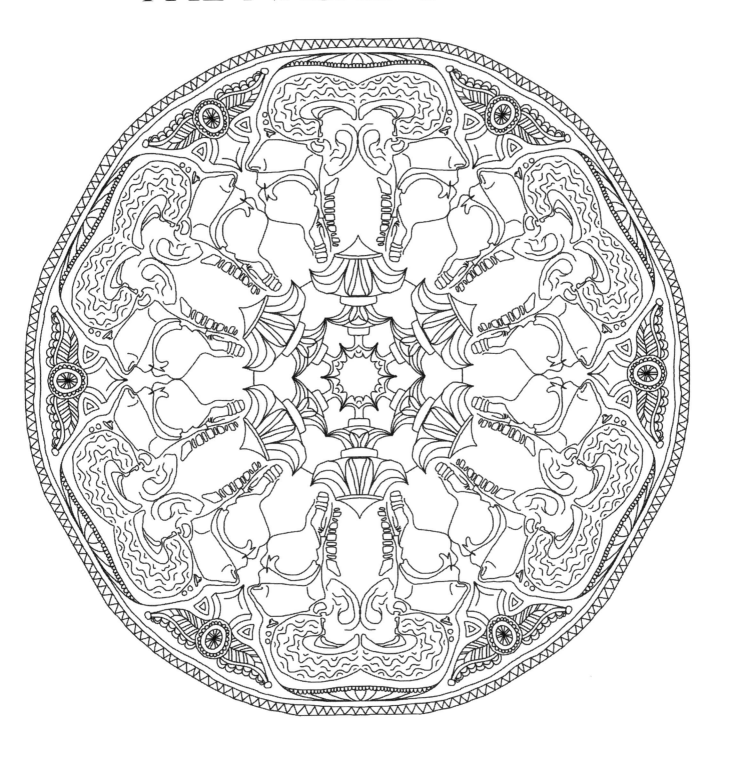

Sound - The Ear

"Do you know what a magical kingdom is in your ear? A fairy cave leads to an Ali Baba doorway, beyond which the bony little ossicles - Malleus, Incus and Stapes - guard the great snail, Cochlea, to whom God has given the power to transform the indiscernible movement of air into music."

Kristin Chenoweth, A Little Bit Wicked: Life,
Love and Faith in Stages, 2009

Sound waves enter the ear through the outer ear, travel along the ear canal and strike the tympanic membrane like a drum. The vibration of the drum skin are transmitted to the three linked inner ossicles, which magnify the motion of the membrane by twenty fold. The ossicles are connected to the cochlea and it is here that the energy of the sound wave is transformed into a nerve signal. The cochlea achieves this feat because its fluid-filled canals generate a further wave that brushes against thousands of tiny hair cells. These hair cells open even smaller pores, which allow ions in the fluid to pass through and stimulate the fibers of the auditory nerve. As with the other senses, the nerves then carry the impulse to the brain.

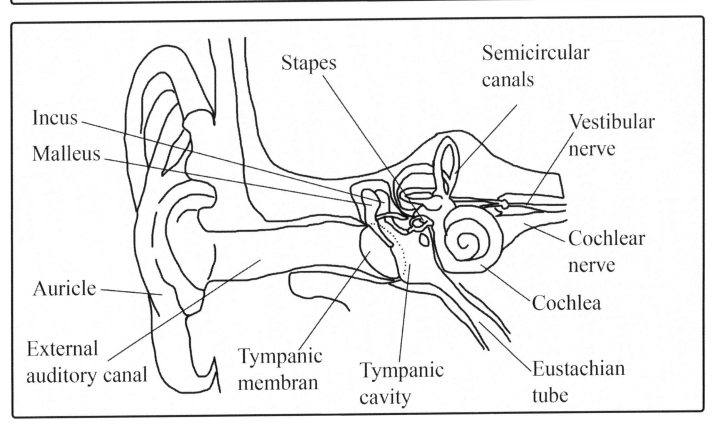

<u>Notes</u>

Color Key:

OUTER EAR: AURICLE, EAR CANAL

MIDDLE EAR: MALLEUS, INCUS, STAPES

INNER EAR: COCHLEAR, SEMI-CIRCULAR CANALS, VESTIBULOCOCHLEAR NERVE

THE EAR

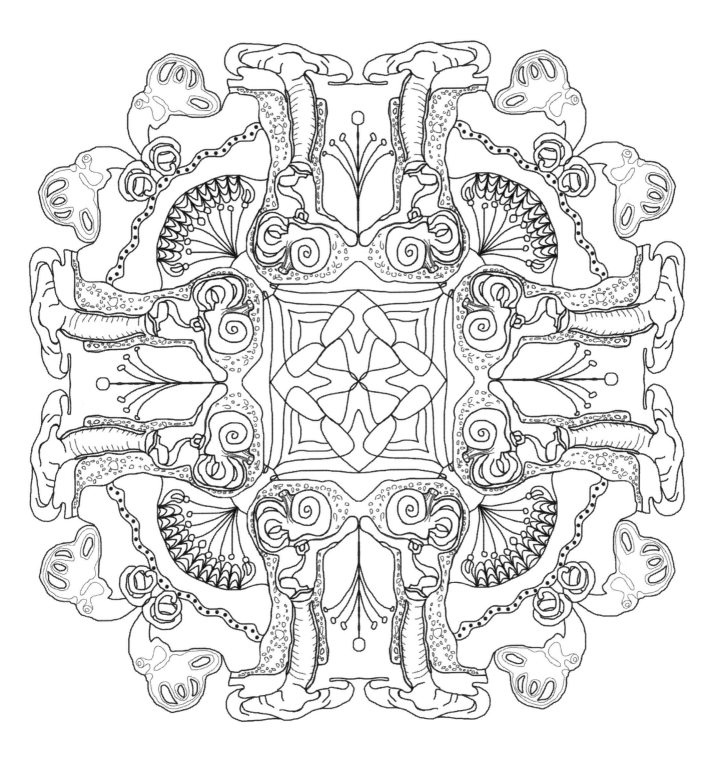

Sight - The Eye

"And now here is my secret, a very simple secret: it is only possible with the heart that one can see rightly; what is essential is invisible to the eye."

Antoine de Saint-Exupury, The Little Prince, 1943

For William Paley, the eye was proof positive of the existence of a supreme designer; for Darwin it was proof of the unstoppable progress of evolution. Such is the anatomical intricacy and beauty of the eye, in its structure and its function, that it remains a subject of discussion across various academic and cultural disciplines. The process of sight is a complex matter of focusing light (itself a complex phenomenon) on to the retina situated at the back of the eyeball. The retina has two types of specialised photoreceptor cells, rods and cones, which change light into electrical impulses that the brain is able to decipher. Rods are able to discern black and white, and are responsible for night vision, whereas cones can detect colours and provide us with detailed vision. The eye actually houses 70% of all the sense receptors in the human body and over a million nerves to transmit the impulses to the brain. It is truly a thing of beauty.

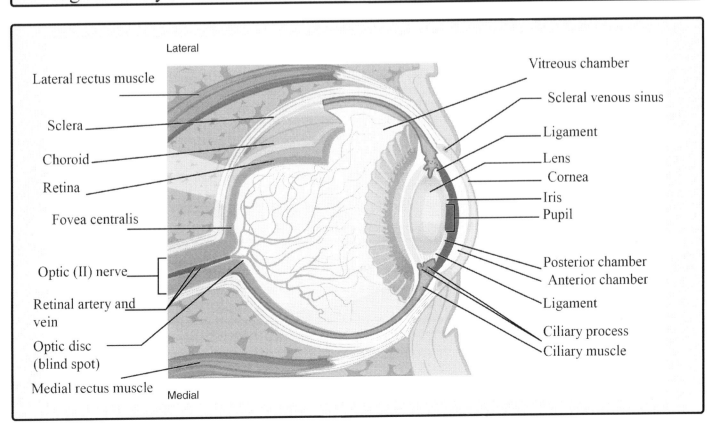

Notes

_____
_____
_____
_____
_____
_____
_____
_____
_____
_____
_____
_____
_____
_____
_____
_____
_____
_____
_____
_____
_____

Color Key:

CORNEA

IRIS

LENS

CILIARY BODY

ORA SERRATA

HYALOID CANAL

RETINA

ARTERY AND VEINS

Sagittal section of the Eye

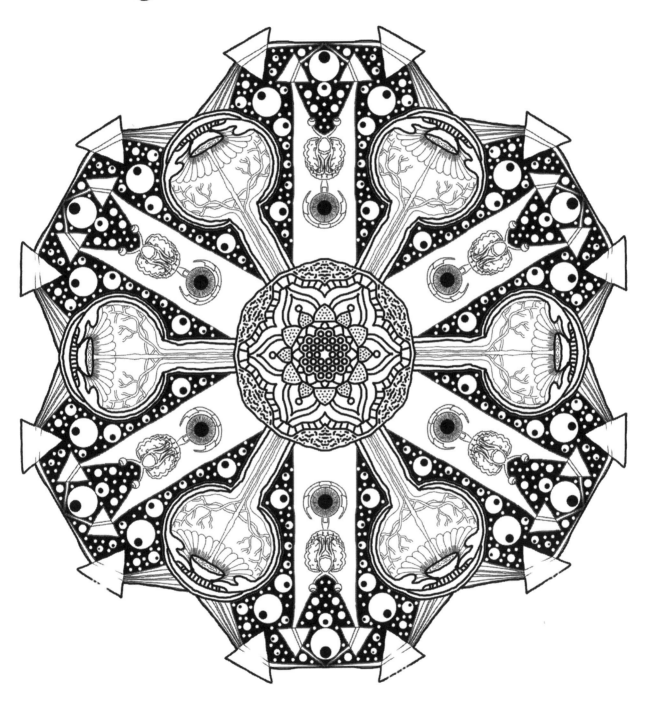

Mitosis

"The science of creating another human is remarkable, and no matter how many times I've learned about cells and mitosis and neural tubes and all the rest that goes into forming a baby, I can't but help think there's a dash of miracle involved, too."

Jodi Picoult, Small Great Things, 2016

Mitosis is the miracle of cell division in which one cell becomes two, two become four, and so on. It is why things are able to grow and heal. The process is divided into five distinct stages:

Interphase - During which the DNA in the cell nucleus is copied and microtubules extend from the centrosomes.

Prophase -The chromosomes condense and pair up, while the nuclear membrane dissolves

Metaphase - The microtubule spindles attach to the chromatid arms of the chromosomes as they line up across the middle of the cell.

Anaphase - The sister chromatids are pulled apart.

Telophase - A membrane forms around each new cluster of chromosomes and two new cells are formed as the original cell divides.

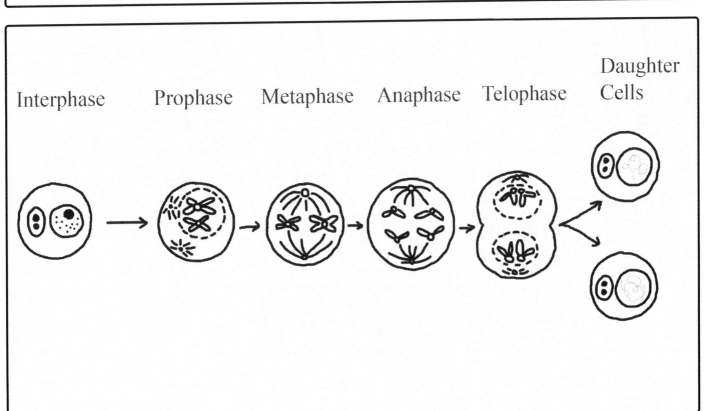

Interphase   Prophase   Metaphase   Anaphase   Telophase   Daughter Cells

Notes

_____

Color Key:
```
INTERPHASE
PROPHASE (X2)
PROMOETAPHASE
METAPHASE
ANAPHASE
TELOPHASE
DAUGHTER CELLS
```

Mitosis

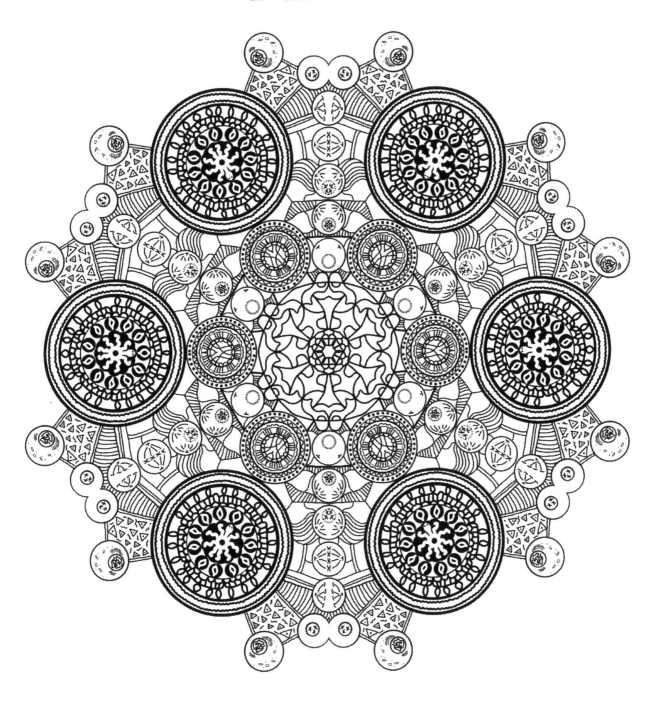

ACKNOWLEDGEMENTS

Many of the anatomical drawings included in this book have been published under a creative commons license. To give just credit to the original artists there follows a list of links at which the images may be found.

Printed in Great Britain
by Amazon